Excuse me, exactly how does that work?

Hocus Pocus in
Holistic Healthcare

Laura Allen

Dedication

To my better half, Champ Allen, who goes days at a time seeing only the back of my head while I'm writing and never complains.

Acknowledgements

Thank you to those people who have shared their knowledge with me over the years, including those people who taught me the things that I no longer believe. It was a part of my journey, and the fact that I didn't interrupt you to ask "Excuse me, exactly *how* does that work?" is not your fault. I don't have anyone to blame but myself for that omission.

Thank you especially to Sandy Fritz, Keith Eric Grant, Bodhi Haraldsson, Paul Ingraham, Whitney Lowe, Christopher Moyer, Alice Sanvito, Ravensara Travillian, Ruth Werner, several mentors that I will not name here, but they know who they are, and all the other people out there who have *made me think*.

Table of Contents

How it All Began

In 1993, I had just opened my third restaurant, *Nothin' Fancy*. Located in the rural community of Greenhill, NC, it was the kind of place that stayed filled with locals, mostly farmers and loggers, and a healthy dose of tourists passing through, since the beautiful attractions of Lake Lure and Chimney Rock are just a few miles up the road.

A nice couple who were transplants from New York started coming in. They had just moved to the area and didn't know many people, and my husband, Champ, and I struck up a friendship with them. Champ actually ended up as a partner in their handmade wooden toy business for a few years, until illness forced him to quit. Hascia was (and still is) a vegetarian, and looked much younger than her years. One day, out of the blue, she asked me if I would go with her to a class called Healing Touch™. At that time, I knew next to nothing of anything about holistic health, and I asked her what it was about. "It's a way of energy healing," Hascia replied. I didn't really know what that was, but I liked Hascia (still do), you had to take a partner, and she offered to pay if I would go. I went.

The class was held at our local community college, and taught by a lady named Jackie. We took turns lying down on the classroom tables, closing our eyes, and running our hands over the bodies of our supine partners and then experiencing them doing the same to us. Whatever we felt was referred to as "energy." We were taught a few techniques for "clearing negative energy" and "balancing the chakras" by "removing the congestion" that exists in the energy field.

I recall placing my hands over Hascia during the class, and I was "feeling her energy." I realize, in retrospect, that what I was feeling was the heat from her body, and my hands were no more than a few inches away from her. There were some nice people in the class, and they all seemed to be into it. I enjoyed the class, which was just an introduction to a longer course of study. Also, I realize, in retrospect, that I never raised my hand and said "Excuse me, exactly *how* does that work?" Neither, as I recall, did anyone else in the class. We were told by the teacher that it worked, and we apparently all blindly accepted that it did.

For the next few years, if someone wasn't feeling well, I would offer them a session. I never charged any money for it, and I don't recall that being discussed at all at the class...whether or not to charge for your "energy work." Maybe they get into that in the advanced classes; I don't know, as I didn't go any further with it.

The people I practiced on were friends and family. I never told anyone it was going to cure them of whatever ailment they had. I usually just said I hoped it would help them feel better. Everyone was always polite about it—they would say it made them feel better—and I'm sure it did help them to feel better, if only for the short term...like most people, we're all caught up in the daily rush called Life, and my recipient would be sitting quietly for at least a few minutes while I "worked" on them. When you're busy, a few minutes of sitting, breathing, and just *being* will definitely make you feel better, won't it? Just sitting quietly for a few minutes is a little break from stress, something we could all benefit from.

One experience that sticks out in my mind happened with Joyce, a woman that I was friends with for close to thirty years, who is now deceased. Joyce had a lot of health problems, both physically, and as the years went by, emotionally and mentally as well. She had been abused during her childhood, then married and had a son when she was just a teenager herself, lived a rather wild life of partying for many years, and had married and divorced numerous times by the time we met through a mutual friend. She had asthma, suffered from chronic respiratory issues but kept on smoking, drank too much alcohol due to self-imposed loneliness, and in her last years suffered severe depression and agoraphobia. I offered her a session one day, and she agreed to have one. Within three minutes of my starting, she was crying hysterically and told me to stop. I did. I never offered again.

More than two decades have passed since I took that class, and a lot has happened since then. I'm no longer in the restaurant business, after more than 20 years of doing that. In 1998, I sold the last restaurant, became a massage therapist, and the rest is history. I want to share some of my journey here. I have hopes that it might inspire some people, and I have no doubt that it will make a lot of people mad, but I'm going to share it anyway. At the very least, I hope it will make some people think, and ask "Excuse me, exactly *how* does that work?" If I have any regrets about switching gears and switching careers, it's my failure to do that when I should have, but I had to go there to get here.

Finding De-Light

This is one of the first magazine articles I ever had published. It appeared in Spirit in the Smokies, a regional publication, in August 1999, while I was attending massage school and graduate school at the same time. I'm reprinting it here, to give you a little insight into where I was at the time.

A number of years ago, I decided something was missing in my life, and set out to find out what that was. I owned a busy restaurant, and I was working on an early death from stress. An acquaintance had read my tarot cards, and told me that I was about to embark on a spiritual journey. As Jerry Garcia said, "what a long, strange trip it's been."

Shortly after the tarot reading, I began meditating each day, outdoors whenever I could, and practicing T'ai Chi. I also began reading the writings of spiritual leaders and mystics, and a lot of pop psychology. I attended my first group therapy session. I started going to a weekly class that studied different things—herbs, Native American practices, all kinds of alternative healing. That group soon evolved into a few of us who wanted to do rather than just to study. Some of my more suspicious friends thought I had joined a coven. We had sweats, animal spirit ceremonies, and went on vision quests.

One of the people in the group started getting colonics, and persuaded me to go. Cleanse the spirit, cleanse the body, she said, so I did. I was also doing a number of herbal purges and treatments. Another friend dragged me to a self-help weekend where I explored my inner child. I started experiencing emotional release, followed by exhaustion. I was attending college at night. One might my professor handed out a blank schedule and said he wanted to know how everyone spent their time for one week. When I finished my schedule, I cried.

Monday through Thursday night, I was going to college classes, and on Friday nights and all day Saturdays and Sundays, I was going to massage school. Tuesday through Friday, part-time, I was working. On Monday I worked another part-time job and attended the weekly meetings of Metaphysics 101. During any odd weekend off, I was always attending a workshop of some sort. Saturday night, the colonic (big party weekend, huh?). Sunday morning, a drum circle; Sunday evening, group therapy. I had one hour left over in my week, and that's the hour I'm at the grocery store and doing my laundry.

In my quest to find spirituality, I had my runes cast, my horoscope charted, talked through a medium to one of my long-departed great aunts, asked the pendulum a thousand questions, attended so many workshops I could conduct my own workshop on "How to do a Workshop." I went through a past-life regression and talked to my spirit guides, and he's what I've found out:

In my quest for spirituality, I allowed myself to become consumed with my mission. I visualized the New Age as the dawning of my time, my time when I was going to leave the old stress-filled me behind, and become a more enlightened, lighter individual. Instead, I jumped on every bandwagon. I didn't stop to consider who the "experts" were that I was listening to. I schedule myself right back onto the same old treadmill I was trying to get off of. I was looking so hard, I got lost.

I've had to lighten up a little. The circle will still keep drumming if I'm not in it. I found out my animal spirit was the Jack Russell terrier who lives next door, and he'll come and see me whether I go to the ceremony or not. The people at group therapy will think I'm having a crisis I don't want to share, but I don't care. I'm stepping back. I'm taking the weekend off, and not attending anything designed to help me. I might go to a baseball game and drink a beer. I'm going to sleep late, and cancel my Saturday night colonic for an old move and a tub of Haagen-Daz. I feel more in tune with my spirituality already!

Onward

I like to think of anything stupid I've done as a learning experience. It makes me feel less stupid.

~P.J. O'Rourke

After selling the restaurant, I got a job as a massage school administrator, and quickly decided I would attend their weekend massage training program for working people. The school was very heavy on energy work. Reiki I was a required part of the curriculum, as was polarity, Traditional Chinese Medicine, reflexology, and several classes that were part of 3-in-1 Concepts (Body, Mind, Spirit), of which the owner was a facilitator.

These involved a lot of muscle testing, and I'm not talking about orthopedic assessments. I'm talking about asking your arms (that was the terminology) if you should eat this or that food, or hire this or that lawyer, or marry this or that person. My husband and I both ended up taking the advanced program in that, which was 120 hours of learning to read people's faces and body language, and giving and receiving a lot of what was referred to as "emotional stress diffusions."

We also went on to do Reiki II, which was optional. That was where we learned how to do distance healing. Yes, I actually believed that you could be in Alaska, and that I could be sitting in my North Carolina home sending you a healing. Again, I was guilty of not raising my hand and asking "Excuse me, exactly how does that work?" A year or so later, we joined the International Association of Reiki Practitioners, and became Reiki Masters in the Usui and Seichim traditions. Champ went on to attend a separate week-long training to become a Gendai Master as well.

The owner of the school collected (and sold) crystals, and used them for healing purposes. I ended up amassing quite a collection of my own, using them to do chakra balances on people, performing psychic surgery with them, and any number of woo procedures. I also purchased magnetic pads for my massage table. I attended homeopathy workshops. I got heavily into essential oils, which I still love and use today—with the caveat that while I think many of them are useful as folk remedies for various simple ailments, I'm not going to advise someone with cancer that they can cure it with an oil, which unbelievably, I notice massage therapists doing all the time—and worse—on social media.

The massage school also had a book store, and I collected every metaphysical book I could get my hands on. I stayed there as the administrator and an instructor for five years after I graduated, and during that period of time, I could not possibly even name all the things I went through. I had a lot of psychic readings. I availed myself of EFT (Emotional Freedom Technique), an invention of Dr. Mercola, which basically consists of tapping on meridian points in order to relieve emotional negativity, food cravings, and pain. I tried Aura Soma, which is described as "color healing." I got tuned up with tuning forks, and crystal bowls.

I participated in one workshop called Matterspeak, which consisted of sitting around chanting random words, letters, and numbers for 8 hours, as in "1263supercalifragilisti789." I don't remember what the purpose of that was and frankly doubt that it had any purpose, other than to enrich the teacher's pocketbook. If memory serves, she had "channeled" that information from the Atlanteans.

I also used the chi machines, the detox foot baths and pads, biofeedback and all kinds of computer programs designed to balance your body, mind and spirit, and most New Agey-sounding things in existence at the time. If it was out there, I tried it.

All kinds of "healers" came and went through the school.

I liked many of these people, the Gendai teacher in particular, who was named Sokari, and was the medicine woman of her tribe in Ghana. She dressed in traditional regalia and was a very regal, imposing woman.

She came over to our house and informed us it was full of bad spirits. She persuaded us to get up and leave before sunrise so she could come in and do a clearing ceremony called Agna Hotra, which we did. The ceremony basically consists of singing a song while burning cow dung throughout the house. When a mutual friend from the massage school came over to our house with her to perform the ceremony, she made the comment "I'm glad you're going to do something about all these spirits in here, they're fucking with you!" "I said "No, they're fine with us, they're fucking with *you*." I'm glad we got that cleared up, because we had been oblivious to the spirits. We still are. Or maybe the ceremony ran them off.

When we were on a road trip out west, I collected some buffalo dung—I actually witnessed the buffalo relieving himself, waited until he ambled off, and I jumped out of the car with a zip-lock bag to harvest it for future ceremonial purposes. Since it had come from a buffalo on the reservation I figured it was more powerful than your average cow dung. I still have it preserved in case the spirits get riled up again and we ever need another ceremony.

I did end up having several spiritual awakenings over the years. And one profound awakening that ended in the Reformation, but I'll explain about that later.

Emotional Meltdown

Emotion is often what we rely upon to carry us across the unfathomable voids in our intelligence.

~Bryant H. McGill

A road-trip out west was the realization of a long-time dream of mine to visit the Pine Ridge Reservation, which is the poorest place in the US—literally. I had been financially supporting the St. Labre Indian School on the reservation since I was a teenager. I took a few weeks off from my job at the massage school, and Champ and I set out to go see it. Before we left, we collected a car load of school supplies for the children. The students and faculty were very generous.

I would encourage everyone in the US to visit Pine Ridge. Located in South Dakota, it's like a third world country within our borders. The average income is less than $4000 a year. Teen suicide is quadruple the national average; suicide overall is twice the national average. Diabetes is 8 times the national average. Cervical cancer is 5 times the national rate. Infant mortality is three times the national rate. The unemployment rate is 80-90%. It has the distinction of having the lowest life expectancy in the US. The only place in the entire Western Hemisphere with lower life expectancy is Haiti.

The US government has placed the Native Americans in a place where the soil won't grow much besides tumbleweeds. Even on the areas that are suitable for agriculture, the money to grow anything is lacking...farm equipment for a family is probably nothing more than a hoe, as any real equipment would be out of the budget. It's so remote, other than an occasional "convenience" store, the closest real grocery or department store is apt to be 100 miles in any direction. Freezing to death is a common occurrence in the winter time. Many of the homes are without running water or sewer.

After we spent the day visiting at the school, which had just been damaged by baseball-sized hail that killed a lot of livestock in the area, we went to Wounded Knee. It's such a sad place, and since it's on the reservation, the government doesn't take care of it. The visitor's center wasn't open, the sign marking the place was so faded it was hard to see the entrance, and the grass looked as if it hadn't been mowed in years.

I sat down in the middle of the cemetery and cried. There were a few other people wandering around. An elderly Native man walked up to me and offered me his tobacco pouch, and told me to take a pinch and cast it to the wind. He said it would soothe my spirit. His presence there beside me soothed my spirit, and I did as he asked. The whole thing was very emotional.

From there we went to the Crazy Horse monument. Chief Arvol Looking Horse happened to be there on the day we visited and I spoke with him for several minutes. Although the monument itself is magnificent, I felt very bad about the circumstances that led to its creation. It is basically a tourist trap, but it is providing employment for a lot of Native people. I had another meltdown while we were there. The very air there just felt oppressive to me, and I didn't want to stay there long. I cried some more as we were leaving. We drove on down to Mt. Rushmore, and I didn't cry at all. It was also an impressive site, but it didn't have any kind of effect on me the way the other places did.

We also visited the Little Bighorn Battlefield in Wyoming, site of Custer's last stand. The statue there has an inscription about how General Custer was sent to rid the territory of hostile Indians, and that just really pissed me off. The contrast between that monument, which is very manicured and cared for by the government, and the one at Wounded Knee, struck me in the heart. There was a guest book in the visitor's center, and I left a nasty diatribe in it about how it was the white people who were hostile, not the Indians. I was crying while I was writing it.

I should qualify my three (so far) crying jags as saying that I am not a crying person. I usually don't even cry when someone close to me dies. It's not that I don't care; I just don't feel that kind of emotion very often, and especially if it was a case of someone who was very sick passing, I usually feel glad that they are out of their pain and misery. I felt a lot of pain and misery of my own on this trip.

The next day, we spent the night in Durango, Colorado. On the morning of September 1, 2001, I woke up in the hotel and flipped on the television. I saw a plane hitting the World Trade Center and thought it was just a movie. In another minute, I realized it was the news. I yelled at Champ to wake up, and we sat there mesmerized for several hours, just stunned and unable to move. We had planned to drive down to Mesa Verde that day, and we decided to go on down there. For the next week, it was very strange driving through the desert not seeing any airplanes or chemtrails in the air, as everything was grounded. We listened to the news on the car radio as we drove along, and in between the sadness at the poverty we were seeing, and the attack on our nation, I just felt raw. I really can't describe it any other way.

A lot of people have the perception that reservations are all prosperous tourist destinations with a casino in the middle that the tribe is getting rich off of. That is a false perception. For one thing, not every reservation has casinos, and on those that do, the majority of them are not getting rich. There are a few tribes where the members are getting really prosperous, but those are the exceptions and not the rule. Many of the casinos employ a majority of non-Natives to the extent that they're not even lowering the unemployment rate at all. Some of the reservations are so spread out that lack of transportation, and lack of money to buy any reliable transportation, keeps the people from being able to go to work at the casino or anywhere else. In many places, the casinos are just making enough money to cover the operating expenses and pay off the debt incurred in building it to start with, and the tribes aren't getting any payout at all.

We ended up visiting a couple of Navajo reservations in Utah and New Mexico, and on the way home, the Cherokee reservation in Oklahoma, which was the most prosperous of all the reservations we went to.

When we set out on this trip, we had only intended to visit the reservation on Pine Ridge and spend the rest of the time playing tourists, but it just kind of snowballed from there and we ended up spending 19 days going from one reservation to another, with a couple of days off to visit my brother while we were in Colorado. It was such an eye-opener. We saw people living in traditional hogans, and many living in the rattletrap government trailers that look like little more than a few sheets of plywood and aluminum siding thrown together. We talked to some of the people everywhere we went. It was a life-changing experience for me, and anytime I worry about money or start to feel like I don't have enough, I try to remember those people who don't have enough food to eat or running water or heat for their homes.

We adopted a family on Pine Ridge. We had good intentions, and the program we went through put us in contact with the family we were supporting. In my ignorance, I wrote a letter to the matriarch of the family, and asked her favorite colors. I had thought about buying her some clothing, and her response to me was "Thank you, but what we need more than anything is food." How about that for a reality check! For the price of a large coffee from Starbucks, these people could eat for a day.

One Christmas, Grandmother (as she encouraged me to call her) asked for a sewing machine. Her old one had just worn out and she told me by making and selling quilts, she could supplement the family income. She was not looking for a handout. She was looking for a hand up. I am glad we were able to provide it.

After we got home from that trip, I got a little further incensed. A tall man dressed in jeans, cowboy boots, and a silver belt buckle walked into the school one day and wanted to speak to the owner. He persuaded her to offer a class in Native American shamanism. I don't know whether he was an actual Native American or not, but let's say I gave him the benefit of a doubt... right up until the moment I heard he had contacted someone I've known for a long time who has a monthly sweat lodge, to ask her how to conduct one. At that point, I figured he was a charlatan. The program cost several thousand dollars and immediately, people signed up for it. I felt that it was a flagrant waste of money, and that anyone who thinks going to a workshop is going to turn them into a shaman is full of shit.

Native American tribal leaders frown on the very term, "shaman." It is not a part of their history, and they don't appreciate people charging money for sweat lodges and vision quests.[1]

I made a list of legitimate Native American charities and started passing around the list and telling people if they *really* wanted to keep Native traditions alive, they should put their money where their mouth is and actually do some good for the people instead of spending their money on a fake shaman. It didn't go over well. I actually left my job at the school shortly after the class started, although that wasn't my reason for leaving.

If you are interested in helping a Native American charity, I can recommend those listed below. They publish their Form 990 finances annually and operate transparently.

Native American Heritage Association spends 94.5% of their collected monies on the programs they administer to the Lakota Sioux, including those on Pine Ridge. Only 1.8% of their collections go toward administrative expenses.

---

[1] **http://www.bluecorncomics.com/stbasics.htm** Accessed 07/10/2014.

First Nations Development Institute works to improve economic conditions for Native Americans through training and education, advocacy and policy, and direct financial grants.

Adopt-a-Native-Elder Program is one of my favorites. Your donations provide food, medicine, clothing, fabric, and yarn to the elders so they can help support themselves.

Taking the Plunge

A friendship founded on business is much better than a business founded on friendship.

~John D. Rockefeller

Five years after I had first come to work and train at the massage school, a co-worker asked me one day if my husband and I could come over that night. She said she and her husband wanted to talk to us about something.

We had actually met these folks while I was still in the restaurant business, when they had purchased some land near our café and started eating there. They had spent years living in the city, and had a dream of running an organic farm. They were so desperate to leave the rat race behind, and didn't have the money to build a house, so they were living on their acreage in a Native American tipi. They were off the grid, and had a neat solar powered outhouse that was a work of art.

They had also formerly been Mormons, although they had left that behind, but they were still adhering to the practice of stockpiling for the future, and they had a shipping container on their land filled with dried food and enough items to sustain themselves in the event of a disaster. My husband later ended up building them a small house/office; those are gaining popularity today as "tiny houses" and they were slowly building their dreams.

The woman of this pair had formerly been an office manager of a medical practice. One day at work, the massage school owner had mentioned to me that she needed office help and I thought of her. She ended up taking the job, and ended up attending massage school as well. Her husband was a freelance television camera operator, who primarily worked sporting events such as basketball games and Nascar races, for which he now had to commute. He also ended up attending the massage school, and taking advanced training in orthopedic massage as well, which he immediately started teaching. We really liked them.

To make a long story short, we went over to their house that night to see what was up. They asked if we had noticed the new professional building that had just gone up in our small town. They had already been down and scoped it out, and wanted us to be their partners in opening a massage clinic there. We discussed it at length over the course of several meetings, and decided to take the plunge.

We actually took two plunges at once. Although Champ has attended massage school and now has a license to practice, which he didn't even try for until he had been out of school for about ten years, massage has never been his priority. He is a carpenter by trade, and that's his passion. He loves to build. Champ had been working for another contractor for a long time, and I had been encouraging him to go out on his own. Our phone rang off the hook with people wanting him to do a job on the side, and I felt sure he would have enough work to do if he just went for it. He decided to do that virtually at the same time we decided to open the office, so we were in the scary position of giving up two guaranteed incomes for an income that wasn't guaranteed at all. It was a definite leap of faith.

We planned to open the office in August. She wanted to keep her job at the massage school until the first of the year, and the plan was that we would be open from 8 am until 8 pm. She vowed that if I would be there from 8am-5pm, that she would come and run the place in the evenings. Most of his camera work was on the weekends, so he had planned to be at the office Monday through Thursday.

I gave my 30-day notice at the school, and offered to train a replacement. On my last day there, the owner gave me a nice going-away party and a beautiful picture as a gift. We parted on good terms, and she actually told me her heart was no longer in running a clinic, which had also been located there, and that she would refer people to me. I was a little surprised, but she did in fact end up doing that.

I really have never been more shocked at anyone's behavior than I was at our new "partners". Almost from day 1, they just weren't there. At that time, we had a little bit of money, and they didn't, so we paid the rent deposits, power deposits, etc., and for their equity in the business, they apparently maxed out a couple of credit cards furnishing the office. I thought it was over the top. It was much more fancy than I had envisioned, but she was having a good time decorating, and I thought well, she's spent five years living in a tipi and now she's in a tiny place that really has no room for decorating, so even though it wasn't to my taste, I just let her go at it full-speed ahead. That was really about the extent of her participation. Within the first week of two of opening the business, she was calling saying she was too tired to come down after working at the massage school all day, and if I didn't feel like staying, to just lock up and leave.

My last restaurant had been open from 5 am until 8 pm, and I was usually there from 4 am until after 9 pm. I had opened that place in a location that I had probably seen ten different owners in and out of over the years, and they all sabotaged themselves by not keeping regular hours...you'd go there for breakfast and find that they might be open at 6 and the next day they wouldn't even be there at 7, and they just closed whenever they took the notion. They all eventually failed.

When I had announced I was opening a restaurant there, a lot of people said "don't go there, that place is jinxed!" I said "No, it is not jinxed. These people have screwed themselves by not being there when they are supposed to be there," so I am just a stickler about keeping regular hours. It didn't work for me to be casual about when we were going to open and close. I felt we were advertising certain hours and that we should be there those hours, but it was pissing me off that they weren't doing their part. Sometimes days went by and I heard nothing from them.

One Monday morning, she came walking in the door. I was surprised to see her because Monday was the day that she and the massage school owner usually spent huddled in the office counting the weekend's proceeds, paying bills, etc. She said that she had realized she was not putting any energy into the clinic, and that she was ready to begin work in earnest, that she had gone ahead and quit her job at the massage school.

Since I had been the one to set up the computer and the filing system, the financial records, and all the other office details, I spent the day showing her where everything was and how it was set up. In my mind, she was there to work from there on out. She didn't come in the next day, or the day after, or the day after that. I never heard a word. Several days later, her husband walked in the door and I went ballistic. He said "I guess we should have told you, but she has decided to stay at the massage school."

I was so mad, I called on Sokari, the Gendai teacher who I viewed at the time as a mentor. She listened to me rant for a while, and then said "What do you want to happen? Do you want them to leave?" I told her yes, I did, that if they weren't going to actually participate in the business, other than to voice an occasional objection about how I was running things, which they were in fact doing, that I wanted them to get out. For example, they didn't want to spend the money to have a listing in the Yellow Pages. Bear in mind, this was 2003, before everyone carried around smartphones or notebooks. Champ and I told them we would pay for it ourselves, although we were supposed to be splitting expenses—and profits, if there were any—equally. They also didn't want to join the Chamber of Commerce, which we felt was important, and again, we said we would pay for that.

I had strong feelings about how to run a good business, and I had been running them since I was 19, which is when I opened my first restaurant. That one was a failure and a learning experience, and the other three were busy places. I felt our clinic could be a busy place, but I also felt we were trapped in some kind of never-never land with partners who were not participating. Sokari said "They know they are not doing right. Just sit back and keep your mouth shut, and I promise you this will all come to a head in a week or two."

She was right on the money. A couple of weeks later, they walked in the door, burst into tears, and told us that they realized they had made a big mistake. They said they could plainly see that this office would never support four people. The announced that they wanted to move to Florida, and that since they had incurred all this credit card debt in furnishing the office, that they were going to have to take out the things that they had paid for and return or sell them, unless we wanted to pay them for all of it. I just smiled and told them my husband would help them carry it out. Not only was it not to my taste, but I had asked them from day one for an accounting of what they had spent, and they didn't want to divulge that. She had finally faxed me a handwritten list of things with prices, and I had responded to that with "The IRS wants to see receipts, and so do I." I never got them.

During this emotional scene, they also stated that they knew they were responsible for half the business expenses for the next three years, which was in the contract we had signed with each other. I let them go out the door thinking that was the case. As soon as they got out the door, I told Champ to give them enough time to go home, and then to call and tell them they were released from all obligations to us.

Champ, who is a nicer person than I am, helped them load all the furnishings on the truck except for a few items that I agreed to buy, and the desk, that they said they would give us for the trouble we had gone through. As they were leaving, he shook hands with them and wished them the best of luck. The man said "You are a funny man." I guess he was expecting Champ to cuss him or something, but if so, he was disappointed. Champ did indeed call later that day and tell them we were releasing them from all contracts, and they were incredulous that we would do that. At that point, I just wanted them gone.

Almost 11 years later, we're still here. We've survived a lot of rough times and economic downturns. We've employed as many as a dozen people at once during those years, although last year, due to the departure of a couple of people we decided not to replace, we have less than that now. I'm at the age and the stage of my career where expanding that business into anything bigger is no longer a part of my plan. We plan to roll on a few more years in the same space with roughly the same amount of people and work our way towards semi-retirement from daily operations. I hope one of my staff members will eventually buy me out so I can focus more time on writing and teaching.

Champ still does carpentry work and a little bit of massage on the side, and sometimes covers the desk at the office when I'm away. We have enjoyed a good reputation in our community, and we're active in our community. We try to support other small businesses and do our part to keep Main Street USA alive. I serve on the board of our local Chamber of Commerce.

I have authored four massage-related books, had dozens of published magazine articles, and have written over 300 blogs. I've been fortunate to get to travel and teach and be involved in the education and the governance of massage. Changing careers during my mid-life crisis has been a great thing for me. I've enjoyed it and I'm still constantly learning. The day I know it all is the day I plan to quit.

Woo on the Menu

It's funny how humans can wrap their mind around things and fit them into their version of reality.

~Rick Riordan

By the time we opened the business Champ and I were both offering reiki sessions. So was the male partner in our business. However, I did want to work with the medical community, so "Energy Work" appeared on our brochure at the very bottom with a little blurb about bring the body into balance and being relaxing...no claims of healing people. Still, I had reservations about putting it on there at all. We did almost immediately start receiving doctor referrals, and not very many calls for energy work, so apparently it went largely unnoticed.

I had received my approval from the **NCBTMB** (National Certification Board for Therapeutic Massage and Bodywork) as a CE provider, and we were also teaching reiki classes.

It's hard for me to explain exactly what happened next, but I literally woke up one day and I was thinking about teaching a reiki class, and all of a sudden I thought, "This is total bullshit. How is my drawing a few symbols in the air and blowing a puff of air onto someone going to turn them into a healer?" A big voice inside my head said "It's not." Call it an epiphany.

That same day, I tore up my Reiki Master certificate. I contacted the NCBTMB and told them to remove it from the list of classes I was authorized to teach. It had to stay on my page there for a period of four years after I had taught the last class. I felt embarrassed about it, but I couldn't do anything about it. I was rather vocal about the fact that I had stopped. I went so far as to apologize to people I had taught and offer them a refund. Most of them thought I had gone crazy, and none of them intended to give up doing reiki on people. I really felt ashamed of myself, and I just kept having the thought that during my own reiki classes, I had never once asked "Excuse me, exactly *how* does that work?" And to top it all off, I cannot ever recall teaching a class where any student of mine questioned it, either. Blind acceptance, people, that's the only excuse I have, just plain blind acceptance.

I have often teased my husband that he has the hottest hands in the universe. Champ will still do a reiki session on someone, if they ask, or sometimes he just offers one to people in pain. I suspect he'd give an attunement if someone asked him to, but we don't discuss that in our house, just like we don't discuss politics. We're on different sides of the political fence, and it will break out into an argument, so we just don't go there. We don't share the same views on religion, either, but somehow, we've been happily married for 21 years. My mother was raised a Southern Baptist and the stepfather who raised me along with her was an atheist, and they didn't argue about it, either. Go figure.

I removed "Energy Work" from our menu of services at the office several years ago. There are a couple of people working there who attended the same massage school that Champ and I attended, and who are perfectly capable of giving a session, but we don't get asked very often. In all fairness to the owner of the school we attended, although she was the queen of woo, she always said we should not perform energy work on people who don't believe in it, don't want it, and haven't asked for it. I respect her for that, and wholeheartedly share that attitude.

Once in a while, someone calls or comes into the office who asks for reiki. I will explain that I don't think it has any basis in reality but can have a strong placebo effect, and I stop with that. When one man came in who asked for reiki, after he shared the details of his aches and pains, I said "Do you mind telling me why you're seeking reiki for that instead of massage?" He told me he had been getting reiki for 15 years and that he loved it, and that he didn't want to take off his clothes. I didn't try to change his mind. I gave him an appointment with someone who still does it.

That is, however, a die-hard rule at my office: *do not do it on people who don't request it.* I had a former staff member that had been with me for six years, and a couple of years ago I was upset when she decided to leave—for about 48 hours.

I had actually figured that a lot of clients would follow her out the door, but her former clients kept dwindling in to our office, in spite of the fact that I know she had contacted her regulars and told them where she was going to work. One man that had never seen anyone else came in, much to my surprise, and I suggested to him that he might want to try several different therapists there to see whom he preferred. He said "Could I just have anybody who won't try to mess with my chi?" I almost spit my water out on him.

Another lady said "I thought she was falling asleep. She would just sit there with her hands on me for a long time and not move." I realized immediately that she was doing energy work on people she had not discussed that with and who didn't want it. My disappointment at her departure quickly evaporated.

The Reformation

*The truth does not change according to
our ability to stomach it.*

~Flannery O'Connor

I'm borrowing that term from Keith Eric Grant. Keith started
out as a Facebook friend, one that I later met in person. He's
one of the people I admire the most in this business. He may
have the distinction of being the only massage therapist in
America who is also a computational physicist and
atmospheric scientist. He is a science writer who has the
ability to explain things to me in terms that my non-scientific
brain can get it. He has also been blogging about the politics of
massage many years longer than I have. Yesterday, I saw he
had made a comment on FB saying that I had joined "the
Reformation." I like it.

About five or six years ago, I got an invitation from Whitney
Lowe to join a forum he had going on, about the evidence-
based practice of massage. I had never even heard the term.
Lord knows I am not known for keeping my mouth shut, but I
sat there for a few months and didn't contribute a word to the
conversation as I watched Whitney, Erik Dalton, Bodhi
Haraldsson, and some of the other Ph.D.'s from the world of
massage discussing EBP. I was gobsmacked. I thought "here is
another way to look at the practice of massage."

Then I chanced to make a few other friends on social media, most of whom I have also now met in person. They are scientists and researchers and educators, and a lot smarter than I am. I am very hopeful that some of that has rubbed off on me, and I think some of it has.

After my rude awakening about reiki, which at the time I learned I had absolutely no scientific basis for believing in to begin with—and at the time I quit practicing it, no scientific evidence for casting it aside, either—I said a few things about it on FB. I immediately inspired the ire of hundreds of massage therapists who do energy work, and got a few complements from the other side for stating my beliefs...I think of it as "the crystal carriers vs. the white coats." I was a member of a bunch of different FB groups where this is argued about all the time, and I would jump right into the fray.

A few months ago, I gave up most of the groups, except for a few that are directed towards EBP and educators. The arguing was wearing me down and I must say, I feel like it's a losing battle to try and impart a different way of thinking to people who are set in their belief systems.

All I can say is that I was once set in mine, as well. Contrary to what people may think, it's hard to do a 360° and not feel a little squeamish about it, especially when you're known to a lot of people. There are magazine articles I've written in years gone by that embarrass me now, but I just can't round up every copy on the planet. I can't retract every conversation I've ever had with anyone on the subject, explaining energy work to them, and I can't undo all the sessions I've done in years gone by.

I've had the thought that some long-ago client may walk in the door one day, and ask me for a chakra balance. Should I say "Sorry, but I don't believe in that anymore."? Should I just give them one for old-time's sake? It's not like I've forgotten how. I can balance chakras with the best of them—if they actually existed.

One of my best-selling books contains three chapters on energy work, specifically Traditional Chinese Medicine, Ayurveda, and the chakras. It's a prep guide for passing the MBLEx and the National Certification Exams, and since those questions appear on the exams, it was a mandate from the publisher that they appear in the book. I have that knowledge, if you want to call it that. In fact, when I took my own licensing exam back in 1999, the only thing available to us at the time was the National Certification Exam in Therapeutic Massage & Bodywork, which included Eastern modalities on the exam.

I remember feeling grateful that I had attended a school that taught all that, because I probably had 25 energy work questions on my exam, and that's a lot of information—whether you believe in it or not—to try and learn by yourself. I remember thinking at the time that I probably had an upper hand over students who hadn't had any schooling in it.

Although I have personally been told by someone at the NCBTMB that they had decided to take a more "Western approach" with their exams, they still list reiki and shiatsu as modalities one may be tested on in the Candidate Handbook. The MBLEx breakdown uses the term "energy anatomy" on their breakdown as well. It seems to be firmly entrenched, to the dismay of evidence-based practitioners.

Faith-Based vs. Science-Based

Far from being demeaning to human spiritual values, scientific rationalism is the crowning glory of the human spirit.

~Richard Dawkins

I'm not one of those people who must have a scientific explanation for everything in the universe. There are things that have not been explained and may never be explained. There's no double-blind study we can conduct to prove the existence of God, for example. Believing in the existence of God is taking something on faith. It's a spiritual or religious belief that is faith-based, and that you are certainly entitled to if you choose to believe. It is not science-based.

To me, that perfectly describes energy work, because there is a lack of any scientific proof that it works beyond anything other than the placebo effect, and there is plenty of scientific proof that it violates known physical laws of the universe. It's something you're taking on faith. As a friend of mine, Dr. Christopher Moyer, eloquently stated in a video he did about reiki research[2], you can't separate the fact that someone who is receiving reiki is having a social visit with a compassionate person who is offering them non-sexual, non-threatening, non-judgmental touch, from the supposed effects of reiki.

[2] **https://www.youtube.com/watch?v=bgkJhFlfO60** Accessed 07/01/2014.

Laying on of hands was something I witnessed in several different denominations of churches as a child. Anyone who was ill could come up to the altar, and people would encircle them and put their hands on them while imploring God to heal them of their ailment. Did it heal them? I don't know, as I was a child and I've never seen most of them again, but I don't have any doubts that it may have made them feel better, at least temporarily, to be surrounded by a bunch of concerned people laying their hands on them in a compassionate way and praying for them.

In any hospital in America, at any given time, there are ministers and chaplains walking into hospital rooms and offering people their prayers for a successful surgery or a speedy healing. I've experienced it myself when I was in the hospital. I've never been asked to pay for that service. In every church I've ever been in, the collection plate has been passed around, but I've never seen anyone thrown out of church for not putting in money. Since faith healing is based on that same type of faith—believing in something that there is no proof of, and which one can't see, is it truly right to charge for that type of service? There are plenty of people making a living doing it.

I'm appalled at the number of massage therapists—and others—who will introduce themselves as healers. I just want to gag, and I've felt that way since long before my Reformation. They honestly believe they are helping people. And when I was doing it, I honestly believed it, too.

I've given many people the impression that I am dead set against energy work. That isn't true. I'm just dead set against holding it out as something other than what it is—faith-based, belief-based, spiritually-based, or however you want to say it.

If an energy worker said "I'll be glad to perform this treatment on you...it's a form of faith healing. There's much scientific evidence that it doesn't work, at least not in the way that I claim it works, but I believe in it anyway and it's something I take on faith, so I'll be glad to perform it if you want me to, and it will be $75..." I could agree with that, but who is going to make such a speech? No one that I know!

I still occasionally lay hands on people, usually if they are ill, in the hospital, and beyond the point of receiving massage. I just no longer have some wild story to go along with it, and I don't charge anyone money for it. I think if you lay your hands on someone with the intent to calm them, soothe them, comfort them, or ease their passing, that intent will be evident in your touch—the same evidence that would be there if you slapped someone hard in the face. Your *intent* to do harm would show, wouldn't it? Why wouldn't your intent to be comforting and compassionate to someone show? Of course it will.

The last time I laid on hands was a year or two ago when my cousin was dying. I visited him in the hospital the night before his passing and asked if I could lay hands on him. My intention was to give him some compassionate touch, and that's all it was. I didn't claim to be channeling any energy from some unknown source in the universe, taking any of his, or giving him any of mine. It was just meant as a comforting gesture.

Something to Believe In

I did then what I knew then.
Now that I know better, I do better.

~Maya Angelou

People like to have something to believe in, don't they? Whether it's religion, the tooth fairy, or the efficacy of something they have bought—and bought into—people get attached to their BS. I like to say that BS can stand for "belief system" or "bullshit"—your call.

Massage therapists, and others in the holistic arts, are no exception. We seem to be a particularly gullible bunch. And there are a lot of people who have seized upon that, and marketed their products, their classes, their modalities, and their wild claims to us...and many of us have fallen for it, hook, line and sinker...and unfortunately, gone on to convince our clients to buy into it, as well.

In many of the debates that I have participated in, whether it was about reiki, alkaline water, crystal table mats or whatever, the believer gets extremely upset if anyone questions how it works. Let's get something straight here, once and for all: **Someone asking for an explanation of how something works is not a personal attack on your character. It's a valid question.** The burden of proof is on the person making the claim, not vice versa! If you're trying to sell something to someone, whether it's a treatment or a product, then you need to be able to supply an answer.

To the people who have said to me "you don't know what you're talking about...if you've never experienced _____," I believe I cleared that up in the first few pages of this book. I *have* experienced it. I've experienced enough to last me a lifetime. I'm not standing here criticizing something that I know nothing about and have never done. I am coming from the perspective of someone who has been there; done that, so don't bother taking that argument with me. It's totally false. I'm liable to try something new today, no matter how hokey it sounds, just so I can say I've tested it for myself. I believe if I'm going to criticize something that should know what I'm talking about.

Our profession has turned into the snake oil medicine show. What if you walked into the drugstore and right inside the door, there's a man on a pedestal selling bracelets. He says "Buy this bracelet, and never take it off, and you will be protected from ever having cancer for the rest of your life! Get one now! It's only $299!" Would you just pay the $299 and accept that, or would you say ""Excuse me, exactly *how* does that work?" If, after hearing his explanation, you felt compelled to pay the $299 and buy it, then you were obviously satisfied with the explanation he gave.

That's what the skeptics are asking for—an explanation. A request for an explanation is not the same as yelling "Liar, liar, pants on fire!" in front of all your FB friends, and yet, the majority of people who are asked for an explanation take it that way.

The arguments from those making the claims are often so ludicrous, they can be picked apart by a high school biology student, much less by a real scientist. Some of the most popular arguments are "it's been around for 5000 years!" So has contaminated water, but you don't want to drink it, do you?

Another popular argument is "This is so advanced; technology just hasn't caught up to it yet." Really? We have landed on the moon and on Mars. We can communicate with telescopes that are hundreds of thousands of miles away from earth. We can predict earthquakes and tsunamis before they happen. We can find miniscule cells of cancer before they blossom into something big. Robots can perform surgery or vacuum your house or defuse a bomb. We can see in the dark and send off remote controlled weapons to obliterate our enemies. We can break apart atoms. We can implant microchips in people and animals. We can use a cheap cell phone as a GPS. We have electric cars. We can send vehicles to the far throes of the planets and the deepest parts of the ocean. We can survive environments that we wouldn't have been able to survive in 100 years ago. The "technology hasn't caught up" argument is looking paler all the time.

The list of faulty arguments on Wikipedia is mind-blowing. [3]T here seems to be no end to it. I'm just picking out a few of my favorites that I see all the time on FB—and that I've been guilty of using myself. I'm trying to do better.

---

[3] **http://en.wikipedia.org/wiki/List_of_fallacies** Accessed 07/01/2014.

Argument from ignorance: assuming that a claim is true because it has not or cannot be proven false. (Again, the burden of proof is on the person making the claim.)

Argument from silence: where the conclusion is based on the absence of evidence, rather than the existence of evidence.

Ad hominem: My personal favorite from FB groups, evading the actual topic at hand by attacking your opponent instead of answering the question.

Appeal to tradition: Asserting that something is true just because it has long been held out as truth.

Begging the question: using the conclusion of the argument as a premise for it.

There are dozens more. Look them up and then ask yourself how many you have used to defend your position. And then answer the real question: "Excuse me, exactly *how* does that work?"

Some of the things that are grounded in antiquity are theories that at the time they were developed, the technology did not exist to dispute them. Take meridian theory, which is the basis for Traditional Chinese Medicine, including the practice of acupuncture.

I'm not even going to go in depth on acupuncture here, because that's another whole book in itself. Research has shown mixed results on the efficacy of acupuncture. Meta-analyses have been compiled that demonstrate that acupuncture is effective, but have plenty of critics, as many of the studies included in the meta-analyses were lacking in strict scientific controls and can therefore indicate nothing more than placebo effect. There is also evidence that sham – acupuncture—needling non-points—is just as effective in controlling pain as acupuncture—meaning that doubt is cast on the validity of specific points and meridians, while supporting the act of needling itself. [4]

In the simplest of explanations, the belief is that a meridian is an "energy pathway." We do have the technology to detect energy—even very minute amounts of energy—that did not exist whenever meridian theory was developed. The same goes for chakras.

If we can detect the energy pulses from stars that are millions of light-years away, don't you think we could detect energy directly flowing through or emanating from the human body? Especially since people are claiming to detect it with nothing more than their human hands? Do you ever realize how incredulous that sounds?

There's more to come about gullibility later in this book, when I'll dissect some of the things we've been particularly gullible to—and that we have passed on to our gullible clients.

---

[4] http://www.ncbi.nlm.nih.gov/pubmed/19250001 Accessed 07/09/2014.

What is Energy, Anyway?

Be able to defend your arguments
in a rational way.
Otherwise, all you have is opinion.

~Marilyn vos Savant

Well, we don't know, at least not in the sense that energy workers speak of it. There is no scientific explanation and no real definition. Some of the claims that are made are that energy equates to "spirit." In a friendly little debate I had with someone who is a big pro-energy believer just last week, my response to his argument was that he was equating energy with emotion.

Bodyworkers often begin a session with "clearing someone's negative energy." I maintain that I can affect your energy, either way, in mere minutes, or even seconds, through my treatment of you. Example: you arrive for your massage right after you've had a fight with your spouse. You're red in the face, frowning, and seething with anger and hurt feelings at the way you've been treated. I greet you at the door with a smile, and say "Leave your stress right here. You can pick it up on the way out, if you still want to." As soon as you're on the table, I start to administer a compassionate touch. Your breathing starts to slow down. Your shoulders start to drop towards the table. You're relaxing, in spite of the mood you're in. I have just affected your energy, wouldn't you agree?

Let's turn that around and say you're in a great mood and really looking forward to your massage. You walk in the door and I immediately start yelling at you, "You're late for your appointment again and I've had it! The world does not revolve around you! I'm sick and tired of the way you treat me like your slave and I am firing you as a client! Don't ever come here again!" I have just affected your energy, wouldn't you agree? Your good mood just ended, and you stomp out the door mad at me and upset that now you have to go to the hassle of finding some other massage therapist who will put up with your constantly being late and still be gracious about it. We can manipulate someone's "emotions" by the way we interact with them. A loving touch will evoke a similar response. A violent slap will evoke fear and anger. So yes, if we're equating energy to emotion, we can all certainly manipulate that.

Some people use the term "subtle energy" to describe the "life force," "chi," "prana" or whatever you're trying to describe.

Medical personnel can usually tell within minutes when a sick person is going to die (as opposed to a sudden death like a heart attack), because life—you could say the life force—wanes in a measurable way, at least at the end of a long illness. The vital organs start shutting down, the blood pressure drops and respiration slows. My own father-in-law passed away one Thanksgiving Day while the family was at his house for dinner. He had been under Hospice care at home, and the nurse stepped into the dining room and announced that he had about ten more minutes to live for those of us who wanted to come in and say our final goodbyes. She was right on the money. Ten minutes later, he drew his last breath.

Even as lay people, we may look at someone we haven't seen in a while, say an elderly grandparent, and think they look grey, or sickly, or whatever, and think "they don't have much time left." It's not rocket science, and it's not magic. There are a lot of clues. And yet, many people want to hang onto supernatural theories. It's their belief system, and once you believe in something, it's hard to give it up—even in the face of reason.

Science has a lot of explanations regarding energy, but to make a long story short, according to Wikipedia, energy is a property of objects, transferable among them via fundamental interactions, which can be converted in form but not created nor destroyed.[5] Work and heat are two processes that can transfer energy. As I stated on the first page about my experience with Healing Touch™, I now know that the "energy" I was feeling was the heat emanating from my friend's body.

There are other forms of energy. We get radiant energy from the sun. We get geothermal energy from within the earth. We can generate electric energy by taking a fossil fuel and converting that potential energy to electricity. Chemical reactions can generate energy.

When reiki practitioners refer to channeling "universal energy," what are they talking about? Nobody knows. They can't explain that, or prove that it exists, but yet, they claim to be "channeling" it. Again, the burden of proof is on the one making the claim, not the person who asks "Excuse me, exactly *how* does that work?" What do you say to clients? How about "I have the supernatural ability to harvest the as-yet

5 **http://en.wikipedia.org/wiki/Energy** Accessed 07/01/2014.

undiscovered energy of the universe and transfer that to you." That's about as honest as it gets.

There are three laws governing energy. Together, these laws form the foundation of modern science.[6] They are:

(1) Energy can neither be created nor destroyed. This means that you can't make energy out of nothing— the total amount of energy in the universe is a constant. (Please note that this applies to a closed system – the Earth is not a closed system, the Earth receives energy all the time from the Sun).

(2) The second law refers to the state of energy and is reflected in a measurement of the degree of disorder, (a measurement called entropy). When you burn a lump of coal, (a material in a very ordered state) a change occurs which results in a more disordered state and you can never combine the resultant products, (heat, gases, etc.) back to form that original lump of coal, (First Law).

The universe, according to scientific evidence, is winding down; the sun will eventually go out, (in billions of years so we don't have to worry right now). In summary when we use an energy source it is not destroyed but enters a more disordered state. This makes the energy less available to us and in converting the energy to power means some loss.

(3)As we mentioned the universe is winding down. The third law is that everything does come to a stop only when the temperature is at −273.15°C on the scale. This equates to

[6] **http://powerplug-in.com/the-three-laws-of-energy/** Accessed 07/04/2014.

−459.67°F. This is called absolute zero and is where the entropy measurement is 0, (Zero).

These laws are absolute physical laws – everything in the observable universe is subject to them. Like time or gravity, nothing in the universe is exempt from these laws. I'm just unclear whether energy workers either have a) no knowledge of these laws or b) they have decided that they are just so special, a universal law about energy doesn't apply to *them*.

So what is it we're about claiming about energy again? And why would we expect people to believe it? Because most people who are not scientists don't understand the physical workings of the universe, people will buy into something...especially when it is someone they look up to as an authority figure, who is spilling the beans on the *real* truth about the universe.

When applied to humans, we need "energy" in order to stay alive. We get that energy from food, along with the oxygen necessary to metabolize it in our bodies. Take away our food, and we will eventually waste away. Take away our oxygen, and we will perish a lot sooner. We can manipulate someone's energy by withholding nourishment from them. We can manipulate someone's energy by withholding oxygen from them. How much sense does it really make to think we can manipulate it by waving our hands in the air above their bodies, or laying a hand on their body? Unless you're laying your hands over their nose and mouth so that they can't breathe, not very much.

So just to recap, we don't know exactly what it is we're calling energy, or subtle energy, or life force, or chi, or whatever. We don't know exactly where it comes from, and we have no idea where it goes when we "clear" it. If you "clear" someone's negative energy, where is that negative energy going? Remember, according to the known physical laws of the universe, it has not been destroyed; it's been transformed. Has it been transformed into positive energy? How can you tell? Is it just hanging around in the ethers ready to zap the next unsuspecting person who walks by with a big dose of bad energy, or would it zap them with good energy, since it has been transformed? Is it landing on the treatment room floor? How are you going to get rid of it? Mop it up? Sage the room and hope it goes up in smoke?

If you are selling or offering something, you need to be able to tell people how it works. If you buy a car, or a new computer, don't you want salesperson you're dealing with to be prepared to answer your questions about it?

I was one of those smart kids in school who loved school and made straight A's. I like to think I'm relatively intelligent. I was a prize pupil, the teacher's pet, and I raised my hand all the time and asked questions. And yet, when it came to this, I failed, and I failed miserably. I didn't raise my hand and say "Excuse me, exactly *how* does that work?" What was I thinking? I guess all I can say is, "I wasn't."

Why Research Matters

Science is simply common sense at its best, that is, rigidly accurate in observation, and merciless to fallacy in logic.

~Thomas Huxley

Research is used to solve problems. It's used to confirm facts, or whatever we think are facts—and sometimes ends up disproving what we thought was fact. It's used to confirm something that has previously been researched. It's used to support existing theories and to develop new ones. It can be used to show that something works, and what efficacy, shortcomings, or ramifications it may have as a treatment. It's used to advance knowledge.

I will borrow again from the words of Keith Eric Grant:

"In disciplined science, one doesn't prove that something does not work. It is the burden of those who claim something does work to prove that it does and with both statistical significance and clinical significance. The "fraud" comes in the implication to lay persons that such significance has been concluded and verified when it is still very much a debatable matter."

One research study is not enough to prove or disprove a theory. Research is meant to be replicated, meaning that if you perform the same experiment someone else has performed under the same conditions, you should get the same results.

Experimental research usually involves direct or indirect observation of the researched subject(s), e.g., in the laboratory or in the field, documents the methodology, results, and conclusions of an experiment or set of experiments.

One well-known study is the *Rosa Study*, named for Emily Rosa, who at the age of 9 became the youngest person to have a study published in the Journal of the American Medical Association.[7]

In 1996, Rosa saw a video of Therapeutic Touch® (TT) practitioners claiming they could feel a "Human Energy Field" (HEF) emanating from a human body and could use their hands to manipulate the HEF in order to diagnose and treat disease. It made such an impression on her; she really wanted to see for herself how it actually worked.

The entire study is **accessible free online from the JAMA.**[8] Here is the abstract from the study:

Context. — Therapeutic Touch® (TT) is a widely used nursing practice rooted in mysticism but alleged to have a scientific basis. Practitioners of TT claim to treat many medical conditions by using their hands to manipulate a "human energy field" perceptible above the patient's skin.

---

[7] **http://en.wikipedia.org/wiki/Emily_Rosa** Accessed 07/03/2014.

[8] **http://jama.jamanetwork.com/article.aspx?articleid=187390** Accessed 07/03/2014.

Objective. — To investigate whether TT practitioners can actually perceive a "human energy field."

Design. — Twenty-one practitioners with TT experience for from 1 to 27 years were tested under blinded conditions to determine whether they could correctly identify which of their hands was closest to the investigator's hand. Placement of the investigator's hand was determined by flipping a coin. Fourteen practitioners were tested 10 times each, and 7 practitioners were tested 20 times each.

Main Outcome Measure. — Practitioners of TT were asked to state whether the investigator's unseen hand hovered above their right hand or their left hand. To show the validity of TT theory, the practitioners should have been able to locate the investigator's hand 100% of the time. A score of 50% would be expected through chance alone.

Results. — Practitioners of TT identified the correct hand in only 123 (44%) of 280 trials, which is close to what would be expected for random chance. There was no significant correlation between the practitioner's score and length of experience ($r=0.23$). The statistical power of this experiment was sufficient to conclude that if TT practitioners could reliably detect a human energy field, the study would have demonstrated this.

Conclusions. — Twenty-one experienced TT practitioners were unable to detect the investigator's "energy field." Their failure to substantiate TT's most fundamental claim is unrefuted evidence that the claims of TT are groundless and that further professional use is unjustified.

THERAPEUTIC TOUCH (TT) is a widely used nursing practice rooted in mysticism but alleged to have a scientific basis. Its practitioners claim to heal or improve many medical problems by manual manipulation of a "human energy field" (HEF) perceptible above the patient's skin. They also claim to detect illnesses and stimulate recuperative powers through their intention to heal.

Therapeutic Touch® practice guides describe 3 basic steps, none of which actually requires touching the patient's body. The first step is centering, in which the practitioner focuses on his or her intent to help the patient. This step resembles meditation and is claimed to benefit the practitioner as well. The second step is assessment, in which the practitioner's hands, from a distance of 5 to 10 cm, sweep over the patient's body from head to feet, "attuning" to the patient's condition by becoming aware of "changes in sensory cues" in the hands. The third step is intervention, in which the practitioner's hands "repattern" the patient's "energy field" by removing "congestion," replenishing depleted areas, and smoothing out ill-flowing areas. The resultant "energy balance" purportedly stems disease and allows the patient's body to heal itself.

To our knowledge, no other objective, quantitative study involving more than a few TT practitioners has been published, and no well-designed study demonstrates any health benefit from TT. These facts, together with our experimental findings, suggest that TT claims are groundless and that further use of TT by health professionals is unjustified.

All touch, if given in the spirit of non-violent, non-judgmental, non-sexual compassion, is therapeutic, isn't' it? Do we really need an incredible (incredulous) story to go with it?

Most massage schools fall short of the mark in teaching their students anything about research literacy. **The Massage Therapy Foundation** has a lot of helpful information on their website and links to other research sites. People sometimes have a fear of even reading research—it conjures up visions of complicated mathematics, and the panic some of us felt as high school or college students trying to write a decent paper—but it's really not that difficult to understand. Believe me, I do not have a scientific mind, and if I can get it, you can get it.

You don't have to be a researcher. You just need to know where to find research, and be able to recognize what makes for a valid test or experiment—as opposed to website hype that many companies post on their page. An endorsement by a celebrity is not a guarantee of any kind that something works. Dr. Oz was recently called on the carpet at a congressional hearing for his endorsement of all kinds of bogus weight-loss treatments.[9]

Randomization is an important facet of valid research. Choosing random subjects for both the test group and the control group of a study, by a computer-generated number system (today's version of drawing numbers from a fishbowl), helps decrease the possibility of bias occurring.[10]

---

[9] **http://www.cnn.com/2014/06/17/health/senate-grills-dr-oz/** Accessed 07/04/2014.

Having a good sample size of test subjects is necessary. Too few, and you won't get an accurate picture. That's one of the reasons Oz was put on the hot-seat—on some of his shows he gave two women the assignment of taking a supplement and then claimed the results were "miraculous" because two people lost a few pounds. Obviously we can't test everyone on the planet, but having too many subjects makes it much more difficult to track results.

The control group in a good experiment receives a placebo, or sham, treatment. Blind experiments conceal information about the test that might influence the tester or the subject. Double-blind experiments conceal information from both tester and subject, an even better way to control bias. Triple-blind is an additional control, when the experiment is monitored by a committee that is not told which group is being tested but is given the data from both groups.

Scientists can be just as attached to their theories as anyone else can be attached to their BS. Studies are sometimes unintentionally biased and unfortunately sometimes fraudulently misrepresented for money, glory, or both. That's why replication is of the utmost importance. One scientist friend of mine said she had a theory, years ago, about something that proved to be wrong. She said "30 years later and I'm still pissed about it!" But she swallowed her pride and wrote up the negative results, which is what should *always* happen. Time spent studying is never wasted, and it's just as much of a service to the public to let them know that

[10] **http://www.uniteforsight.org/global-health-university/research-validity** Accessed 07/03/2014.

something doesn't work, even though you set out to prove that it did.

The Myths of Massage

*The great enemy of the truth is very often not the lie,
deliberate, contrived and dishonest, but the myth,
persistent, persuasive and unrealistic.*

~John F. Kennedy

I like to think I'm a fair person. I would prefer to think well of
people, and give them the benefit of a doubt whenever
possible. I'd like to think that no teacher deliberately sets out
to give people false information. I'd like to think that they are
simply repeating what *they* heard in school, but unfortunately,
when that happens, the next generation of teachers repeats it,
too.

My pet peeve is the toxin myth. I have a **video on YouTube**
in which I talk about toxins [11], and I've gotten a lot of hate mail
over it.

To begin with, what are we calling a toxin? On any given day in
the news, there are stories about toxic water. Toxic air. Toxic
chemtrails. Toxic prescription drugs. Toxic food additives and
toxic genetically modified food. Toxic pollution. Toxin,
schmoxin. It seems that everything around us is a toxin.
Within the human body, though, what are we calling a toxin?

---

[11] **https://www.youtube.com/watch?v=gwTDw1kXpo8** Accessed 07/01/2014.

That word is misused all the time. If you were bitten by a poisonous snake this morning, or had your chemo today, then definitely, you have toxins. Otherwise, you have normal metabolic wastes. We can't squeeze it out of you with a massage. Let's say I spent the morning drinking coffee, dumped a few spoons of aspartame into every cup, had a sandwich with nitrate-filled bacon, smoked a pack of cigarettes for good measure, and then went to get a massage. Is a massage going to squeeze that out of me? No. And yet the standard post-massage speech is "Drink a lot of water for the next couple of days to help flush out your toxins." Excuse me, exactly *how* does that work? Just offer people a glass of water as a courtesy, and skip the toxin speech.

We ought to bear in mind that just because something is a chemical, that does not mean it is a toxin. There are thousands of useful chemicals that are beneficial to humankind, and not toxic at all.

Another myth is that massage will flush out lactic acid, post-exercise. Excuse me, but exactly *how* does that work? In fact, research has not only shown that massage does not flush it out, it is not even the cause of delayed onset muscle soreness, as has been repeated by massage therapists for years.[12] Lactate is used as a fuel, along with carbohydrates and fat. Your heart muscle likes to consume lactate as a fuel, so that's a good thing to have around. If your muscles did not produce large amounts of lactate, they would actually fatigue much sooner.[13]

---

[12] **http://www.ncbi.nlm.nih.gov/pubmed/23256711** Accessed 07/04/2014.

[13] **http://running.competitor.com/2010/01/training/the-lactic-acidmyths_7938** Accessed 07/01/2014.

How about refusing to massage women during the first trimester lest you cause a miscarriage? Do women stop working during the first trimester? Do they stop playing with their children, exercising, or having sex? No, they don't, and unless the doctor has diagnosed some problem with the pregnancy and advised against it, there is absolutely no reason to avoid getting a massage. It would be common sense not to be Rolfing anyone on the abs during pregnancy.

Then we've got the "don't touch the medial malleolus of a pregnant woman, unless she's at her due date, because you could cause a miscarriage." There is no scientific evidence whatsoever that there is any connection between that area of the body and the uterus, and no reason not to touch it. That is a theory popularized by reflexologists. It's more likely that a Martian will beam down and cause a miscarriage than to believe that you are going to cause one by touching someone's ankle.

While we're on the subject of reflexology, which in the past I have availed myself of many times, there is no proof anywhere in existence that there is a corresponding organ to any point on the feet.[14]

I love a good foot massage. Nothing feels better! But is it affecting my gall bladder, my liver, my heart? Excuse me, exactly *how* does that work? If there was in fact a nerve running from the gall bladder to a "reflex point" on the foot, a nerve conduction test would prove that. If there was an electrical pathway, or some other physical phenomenon leading from a point on the foot to a specific organ, we now

[14] http://www.ncahf.org/articles/o-r/reflexology.html Accessed 07/01/2014.

have the technology to detect that, which did not exist when reflexology theory was developed. Another case of "just because it's old doesn't mean it's the truth." Give a great foot massage, and take pride in doing so. That is all.

People look up to their health care providers as authority figures, whether that person is an MD or a holistic practitioner. They count on us to know what we're talking about. That goes double if said practitioner is an educator. Are your clients and/or your students paying you to give them accurate information?

There are so many things out there that just don't have any evidence to back them up. If you're going to make a claim, shouldn't you *have* some evidence to support it? Again, just because a theory has been around for a long time doesn't make it so. People used to believe the earth was flat. Remember that.

It's not a pleasant process to examine ourselves...to take one of those searching and fearless personal inventories. It's not a pleasant process to realize that something we have believed in, and have repeated to others, especially if we charged them money for it, is wrong.

It's not a pleasant process to admit to ourselves, and certainly not pleasant to admit to others, that our belief system is based on ideas that are in direct contrast to known physical laws of physics, chemistry, biology, anatomy, and physiology. The funny thing about that is that some folks who are actually teachers of anatomy and physiology, and *know* how the body works, still teach other things that don't mesh with that at all.

If you're well-known in your field, it's even more unpleasant to have to back up and say "I used to believe this, but now I know the evidence says that it's not so." As I stated earlier, there are things that have not yet been proven and may never be proven, but when there is overwhelming direct evidence to the contrary, I personally can no longer in good conscience ignore that. I can't act like the laws of the universe don't apply to *me*. I'm not that special.

It's been difficult for me for the past few years. I get a lot of criticism for being outspoken about evidence and about asking others for evidence to back up the claims they're making. Just the other day after I shared a research article on my social media, someone immediately chimed in with "I hate to see a prominent teacher that I used to admire and respect slamming alternative health care methods."

After I made an announcement about this book, I saw a post that said "that's one book I won't be buying. It's very obvious that she doesn't believe in miracles." Look at the Wikipedia definition of "miracle":[15]

....an event not ascribable to human power or the laws of nature and consequently attributed to a supernatural, especially divine, agency.[1] Such an event may be attributed to a miracle worker, saint, or faith based leader. A miracle is when a being with supernatural powers, such as a god, works with the laws of nature to perform what are miracles.[2] Theologians say that, with divine providence, theistic gods regularly work through created nature yet are free to work without, above, or against it as well.[3]

The word "miracle" is often used to characterize any beneficial event that is statistically unlikely but not contrary to the laws

---

[15] **http://en.wikipedia.org/wiki/Miracle** Accessed 07/10/2014.

of nature, such as surviving a natural disaster, or simply a "wonderful" occurrence, regardless of likelihood, such as a birth. Other miracles might be: survival of an illness diagnosed as terminal, escaping a life-threatening situation or 'beating the odds'. Some coincidences may be seen as miracles.[4]

That's what I've said: supernatural, faith based.

There are people that avoid me altogether, or that want to argue with me along the lines of "but don't you think that as long as it makes them feel better, it's okay?"

The placebo effect is a powerful thing. It's estimated that 1 out of every 3 people will experience the placebo effect. [16]Just be honest and upfront about the fact that you are doing, teaching, or selling something that is totally based on faith, due to the fact that the evidence against it far exceeds any evidence supporting it, and that any positive effects realized from it are in all likelihood the placebo effect.

We've also got to account for the "expectation effect," meaning if someone expects something good or bad to happen, it's likely to...if they expect to feel better, that's a big possibility, and if they expect to feel ill, that's a big possibility, too. We've all seen that one in action! Let's say two new clients both suffer from fibromyalgia. One comes in the door smiling and says "I'm so grateful, Dr. Reed sent me over here and he said this was really going to help me feel better." The other one comes in looking pitiful and whines "I know this isn't really going to help, but Dr. Reed wanted me to come." Which one of those

---

[16]**http://www.cancer.org/treatment/treatmentsandsideeffects/treatmenttypes/placebo-effect** Accessed 07/08/2014.

people is going to feel better? One of them decided not to feel better before she ever got in the door. It's not rocket science.

Make it very clear to people that what you do is not a substitute for medical care, and encourage people to seek medical care for any potentially serious issues.

First Do No Harm

It is possible in medicine, even when you intend to do good, to do harm instead. That is why science thrives on actively encouraging criticism rather than stifling it.

~Richard Dawkins

Many practitioners may also ask "What's the harm? Is my doing energy work (or homeopathy or crystal healing or whatever) going to actually hurt someone?" No, it isn't—unless the client falls into the trap of believing that you, whom they view as an authority figure, are providing an appropriate substitute for the real medical care that they actually should be receiving, which happens more often than you think. There is a power differential inherent in every therapeutic relationship, and it's in our favor.

When I was a brand-new therapist, I had just started a massage on a woman who suddenly whipped back the drape, and she actually had taped a feminine napkin to her breast. Instantly a rank smell hit me in the face. She pulled back the napkin and said "What do you think of this?" It was an open, oozing wound. I immediately took my hands off her and asked if she had been seen by a doctor. She said no. I asked how long it had been there. She said about nine months. I told her that I could not massage her, and that my strong suggestion was that she leave my office and go immediately to the doctor. She told me she had been to a couple of different energy work practitioners and a naturopath—none of whom suggested that she needed to see a physician. She had been using aromatherapy oils on it. She was in total denial that she had a serious condition.

Her husband was in the lobby waiting for her. I went out and in no uncertain terms told him that he should immediately take her to the emergency room. Yes, I probably was overstepping boundaries, but I was very concerned for this woman and I could not imagine that any hospital wouldn't admit her on the spot. A few hours later, she called back to the office and stated that she had gotten an appointment with Dr. So-and-So on a date that was several weeks in the future. It so happened that my sister-in-law was the office manager there, and I called her and begged her to move the appointment ahead as soon as possible, that I thought it was a matter of life and death. They moved her appointment, but it didn't do any good. Less than two weeks later, her husband called the clinic and thanked me for being so severe with her, but it was already too late. She had Stage IV breast cancer, and she had died the day before. If she had gone to the doctor when she first became aware of the problem, she might still be here today.

Several years ago, a naturopath who practiced about an hour away from my town was sent to prison for advising the parents of a diabetic child to ignore their child's insulin prescription and follow *his* protocol, and the child died.[17] Naturopaths are not licensed in my state—and even if they were, there's no guarantee that the outcome would have been any different.

---

[17] **http://www.quackwatch.org/11Ind/perry.html** Accessed 07/01/2014.

In another case in Oregon, a 53-year-old woman died due to chelation therapy administered by a licensed naturopath, supposedly to "cleanse her of heavy metals." Instead, the procedure sent her into a severe hypocalcemia—a dangerously rapid lowering of blood calcium levels.[18]

We are not doctors. We are not nutritionists, dieticians, psychologists, or any other licensed profession, unless you are actually licensed in that profession. I've noticed a trend of a lot of massage therapists getting themselves "certified" as "health coaches" and that's just plain scary to me.

If, as a health coach, you are cheerleading people into sticking with their diet and/or exercise plan, and helping them to stay motivated to lose weight or otherwise get healthy, that's just dandy, but I am fearful that many people go way beyond that, and this is a relatively new and unregulated field with varying types and amounts of education. Spending a weekend in a CE class does not, in my opinion, suddenly qualify you to be a health coach. Some programs are longer, but in the general scheme of things, they are certainly no match for the type of education required to get in to a licensed profession.

I've also noticed that many of these health coaches are also selling some multi-level-marketing juice, supplement, shakes, powders, or whatever. That alone is enough to keep me away from one, due to the huge conflict of interest that entails. If your coaching practice is a means to get people to buy whatever it is you're selling, you have apparently missed out

---

[18] http://www.sciencebasedmedicine.org/another-state-promotes-the-pseudoscientific-cult-that-is-naturopathic-medicine-part-2/ Accessed 07/01/2014.

on reading the Code of Ethics, which states that we should not take financial advantage of a client for our own personal gain, over and above our normal and customary fee.

It is that kind of attitude that I find disturbing at best, and dangerous at worst. A health coach is not a doctor. A BA is not remotely close to a doctor. Overstepping our scope of practice is a very serious matter that can result in serious harm, or even death, to the very ones we are supposed to be caring for.

Last year, I had pneumonia, which incidentally is the 8th biggest cause of death in the world, and wound up in the hospital for a week. People on FB were telling me all kinds of things I ought to be doing. "You should get Bowen therapy! You should have craniosacral! You need Reiki! You need to do a lung cleanse, and a liver cleanse, and the Master cleanse! You need frankincense!" I even got the comment "If you were on a vegan diet, you wouldn't be having this problem!" The comments looked like a few hundred MTs gone crazy with power, prescribing for me, while in the meantime I'm in the hospital planning my funeral.

Just like any other health care practitioner, our obligation is to *first do no harm.* Giving people advice that we are not qualified to give, and failing to refer someone to a physician when we suspect a serious matter, is a blatant violation of that obligation.

Some will counter with the argument that traditional Western medicine kills people every day. Yes, it does. However, that's another faulty argument—an irrelevant conclusion—where an argument itself may be valid, but does not address the issue in question, which is us overstepping our boundaries.

Hocus Pocus...Caveat emptor

Thinking is the hardest work there is, which is probably the reason why so few people engage in it.

~Henry Ford

How is one to *know* what's bogus and what's not? It's actually a simple thing, called *critical thinking*. Critical thinking means you gather information, evaluate it, analyze it, synthesize it, and apply it. While personal experience may enter into it, so should research. Gathering information from impartial third-party sources is often the missing piece, when it comes to all the marketing hype we're constantly bombarded with. For example, take any product out there...if the only "research" on their website is the claims that are made by the company that is selling the product, that's a big red flag. Further investigation should be the rule of the day, unless you just enjoy throwing away your hard-earned money.

Critical thinking doesn't mean you have to have an advanced degree or be a scientist. It really just means that you have enough common sense to stop and ask "Excuse me, exactly *how* does that work?"

As I stated earlier, massage therapists and other holistic practitioners seem to be especially gullible to wild claims—and in turn, passing them onto their clients. People want to believe in something, and there are a lot of companies out there targeting their marketing to us.

People get caught up in the marketing hype, take the company's word that something works, and suddenly, they're experts in how it's the cure for everything.

In fact, just last night I spent several hours in the emergency room at our local hospital, due to taking a fall on a wet floor. I posted that on my FB page, and immediately, the bombardment started, with my fellow massage therapists saying "You need this! You need that!"

I know people have good intentions, and I truly do appreciate the prayers, and the people saying they are sending me good energy—their heart is in the right place—so I do appreciate people thinking of me and wishing me the best, even by way of those things that are not in my personal BS. I think of that the same way I think of people saying "Merry Christmas." It's a polite greeting, offered in the spirit of kindness, and it's not necessary, in my opinion, to throw that back in someone's face with a diatribe about it being politically incorrect when their intentions are to wish me well.

However, when it goes beyond that, with people telling me I need a $1500 device that has the exact same effect as a $30 heating pad, I beg to differ. I don't care if it's being sold by the President of AMTA or the President of the US. To quote a popular country song, "You've got to stand for something, or you'll fall for anything."

Anything, no matter how strange or unlikely anyone personally thinks it is, is going to have anecdotal evidence...which is the weakest form of evidence on the evidence pyramid. Everyone has their own subjective experiences. We like anecdotal evidence especially when it's personal to us, when we've given someone a massage and they say "I feel so much better, now." It validates us. It flatters us.

However, if anecdotal evidence and testimonials are the only recommendations for the product someone is selling, that's another red flag.

Other red flags to watch out for in a supposedly-health-related marketing campaign [19] include looking at how low-rent their marketing seems to be...if a late-night infomercial on a local station is their sole marketing strategy, that's not a good sign. If the product were that good, they'd have the advertising bucks to spend on prime time television. The word "alternative" is often thrown out there when something hasn't been properly tested or proven to work. Wild promises of "instant" or "miraculous" results suck people in and then fail to deliver. If that kind of wording is in the advertising, run the other way.

Even things that are inherently good can be made to look bad, when media hype, people going outside their scope of practice, and the urge to make wild claims take over. Take aromatherapy, for example.

I think essential oils can be useful for many things. Plants are nature's oldest medicine, and some modern medicines are still derived from them.[20] Many of them have the chemical properties of being antiseptic, antibacterial, analgesic, and so forth.

[19] **http://www.webmd.com/men/features/health-ad-red-flags**
Accessed 07/07/2014.

[20] **http://chemistry.about.com/library/weekly/aa061403a.htm**
Accessed 07/04/2014.

Many essential oil companies (and this is another field that is filled with MLM companies), and people who have virtually never had any training about essential oils, and don't know any more than what's printed on the company website, are guilty of making unproven and downright dangerous claims about their products.

PubMed actually has more than 800 aromatherapy studies indexed.[21] Many of them demonstrate that aromatherapy is useful or at least shows promise for assisting in the treatment of various conditions. In my own review of the first 20 that are listed, the results were mixed. One analysis of various CAM interventions to see if they were effective at reducing agitation in those suffering from dementia showed that aromatherapy and light therapy demonstrated no clinical effectiveness.[22] Another study on whether aromatherapy could reduce anxiety in health care waiting spaces was inconclusive.[23]

One positive study demonstrated that aromatherapy combined with massage could "exert significant influences on multiple neurobiological indices such as EEG pattern, salivary cortisol and plasma BDNF levels as well as psychological assessments."[24] Another study demonstrated that Ayurvedic aromatherapy oils applied during a massage could help relieve

---

[21] http://www.ncbi.nlm.nih.gov/pubmedhealth/PMH0032645/ Accessed 07/07/2014

[22] http://www.ncbi.nlm.nih.gov/pubmed/24947468 Accessed 07/04/2014.

[23] http://www.ncbi.nlm.nih.gov/pubmed/24942321 Accessed 07/04/2014.

[24] http://www.ncbi.nlm.nih.gov/pubmed/24906585 Accessed 07/04/2014.

pain, but had the side effect of causing allergic contact dermatitis.[25]

Another randomized, double-blind study produced positive results in demonstrating that inhaling lemon could substantially reduce nausea and vomiting in pregnant women.[26] One study, conducted on mice, demonstrated that aromatherapy may be useful in relieving stress in humans. [27]

The human olfactory system is a beautiful and complex thing. A certain aroma may remind you of your grandmother's perfume, or your mother's chicken soup, and give you a moment of pleasant memories. Health-wise, though, the wild claims made by aromatherapy companies should be taken with a cup of salt...yes, I know I said "cup" instead of "grain." I mean to emphasize the need for scrutiny. If you read the table mentioned above [28] that lists modern-day medicines that are derived from plants, it's easy to see that none of them were chosen for their fragrant properties. They were chosen for their chemical constituents.

Some people like to perfume themselves with scents that they find pleasant, or diffuse them in a room to enhance their environment. Smells that are pleasing to us may have the effect of making us feel more calm and happy. There's nothing at all wrong with that. And some folk remedies have stood the

---

[25] http://www.ncbi.nlm.nih.gov/pubmed/24891661 Accessed 07/04/2014.

[26] http://www.ncbi.nlm.nih.gov/pubmed/24829772 Accessed 07/04/2014.

[27] http://www.ncbi.nlm.nih.gov/pubmed/24882416 Accessed 07/06/2014.

[28] http://chemistry.about.com/library/weekly/aa061403a.htm Accessed 07/04/2014.

test of time, like peppermint being used to freshen the breath, clove oil relieving the pain of a toothache, and wintergreen or camphor being good topical applications for sore muscles. However, the notion that inhaling aromatherapy oil, applying it topically, or even ingesting it as the cure for all disease is just plain ridiculous, and yet, that's what some would have us to believe.

Many essential oil companies market their blends by giving them names corresponding to emotions or states of mind. For example, one popular company sells "Forgiveness." Is wearing that oil going to cause me to forgive people? Not per se, but it may be a reasonable explanation that every time I get a whiff of it, or someone else says "What's that you're wearing?", I am reminded that there is someone I need to forgive, and I might be more inclined to do it.

Lots of essential oil companies, and in fact, many companies of all kinds that target massage therapists and other holistic practitioners, make the claims that their product will "bring you into balance." Excuse me, exactly how does that work? Are we all out of balance? How do we know we're out of balance? How can we tell when we're back in balance? Is there a balance meter that tells us when we're out and when we're in?

Personally, I love aromatherapy oils, and I own a lot of them from various companies. They in fact do reside in my medicine chest. If I come down with a chest cold, I'll rub some camphor into my chest. I keep a bottle of peppermint beside my massage table in case the client has smelly feet. I put lemon oil in my mop water to make the house smell good.

I have even been a member of one MLM company for close to twenty years. I signed on as a distributor so I could get their products cheaper for my own use. I don't attend any meetings. I don't hold any meetings. I don't try to sign people up for the company, I don't have automatic orders, I don't get checks from the company for recruiting people, and I am not trying to scrape my way up the pyramid ladder to Diamond Platinum Gold status or whatever the latest thing is in their scheme.

There's nothing wrong in using essential oils. Just avoid the urge to prescribe whenever someone mentions an ailment. That is out of our scope of practice, along with diagnosing people, but people are particularly guilty of doing this on social media sites...as soon as someone says they have this or that ailment, including when it's only self-diagnosed and not an actual doctor's opinion, people immediately start chiming in with the oil prescribing. Aromatherapy is an unregulated field in the US, and the training in it varies widely. Being a distributor for some MLM company is not proof of training, and a weekend workshop does not make you an authority on the subject. If you *have* had advanced training in the chemistry of essential oils, and you *do* know what you're talking about, bear in mind that in the US, you are still not allowed to prescribe.

No doubt the few examples of things I've provided below all have anecdotal evidence. People have tried it and liked it, or got something they wanted out of it. Again, that's the power of the placebo effect, or the expectation effect.

A placebo can take the form of a pill, a shot, or any other treatment. They all have one thing in common: *they do not contain any active substance that is meant to affect health.*

People can have positive or negative responses to a placebo. A positive response would be reporting that their symptoms are better, when in fact, nothing was actually done or administered to make them feel better. A negative response, for example, would be experiencing a "side effect" to the treatment, again, when nothing was actually done or administered to make them feel better. Many times, an ailment that just ran its course and went away on its own is probably attributed to faith healing/energy work or other placebo.

I ask, if you are a practitioner, an instructor, or a consumer of any of the items on my sample hit list, to revisit it *with critical thinking*. Put aside your attachment to it. Act as if you are hearing about it for the very first time. Ask yourself the question, excuse me, exactly *how* does that work? If you've been used to explaining to your clients about how it works, do you still feel it's an adequate and truthful explanation?

The consumer has the right to spend their time and money on anything they choose. But if that choice is based on claims that aren't true, that's not an informed choice. *Caveat emptor—let the buyer beware.*

I've listed a few of my personal favorites in alphabetical order, and as I said, it's far from being a complete list; they are just a few of the things that I find the most glaring fault with and that companies spend a lot of money marketing to massage therapists and other holistic practitioners, and that many practitioners turn around and market to the unsuspecting public in general. So much hits the market on an almost daily basis there will probably be 20 new ones before I finish writing this.

Access Bars®

When I first heard of Access Bars®[29], it immediately reminded me of 3-in-1 Concepts training that I took years ago, part of which was about "wiping out genetic memory," purportedly so you don't keep making the same mistakes and same bad life choices. The company is actually called "Access Consciousness®, and Access Bars® is just the first class in their multi-level training, but it's the one that receives the most attention and their marketing focus seems to be on that. Here's part of the hype from their website:

Did you know there are 32 points on your head which, when gently touched, effortlessly and easily release anything that doesn't allow you to receive? These points contain all the thoughts, ideas, beliefs, emotions, and considerations that you have stored in any lifetime. This is an opportunity for you to let go of everything!

Each Access Bars® session can release 5-10 thousand years of limitations in the area of your life that corresponds with the specific Bar being touched. This is an incredibly nurturing and relaxing process, undoing limitation in all aspects of your life that you are willing to change.

Excuse me, exactly *how* does that work?

If these 32 points actually existed, wouldn't there be evidence of that, for example on an MRI or a CAT scan? Then again, who needs any evidence? Not the people practicing this,

[29] **http://www.accessconsciousness.com/classtype_details.asp?cid=11** Accessed 07/02/2014.

apparently. As for the 10,000 years' worth of limitations, I'm really not disturbed by thinking that 10,000 years ago, my ancestors were barefoot, living in a cave, and hunting and gathering food. (In fact, I may still have one or two that are pretty close to living that way). Are we all carrying that around in our psyche like it's some kind of secret shame, and we're supposed to be upset over that to the point that it is affecting our daily lives? Give me a break. Does this "opportunity to let go of everything!" mean that our good memories will be wiped out along with the bad?

The founder, Gary Douglas, was a real estate agent in California who "channeled" this information.

One news article described Douglas thus:

Around the time Douglas's real estate business imploded, he discovered his own channeling powers. One night, his body was taken over by the spirit of Grigori Rasputin, the Russian mystic who was assassinated in 1916. Douglas would later joke about how it was just his luck that he couldn't be a conduit for any of the typical angelic beings claimed by other channels. Douglas didn't entirely trust Rasputin, and he eventually was inhabited by other spirits, including a "wise ancient Chinese man named Tchia Tsin," a "robust, rowdy" 14th-century friar named Brother George, and a group of alien beings called Novian.[30]

Really? Do you want to spend your hard-earned money on this? According to their website, they now have over 2000

---

[30] **http://www.houstonpress.com/2012-11-08/news/gary-douglass-access-consciousness/3/** Accessed 07/03/2014.

facilitators in 47 countries. Sounds like they're making the big bucks. Beam me up, Scotty.

One former participant stated that "Questions, doubt, and dissent are discouraged," and that anyone who didn't agree with the group leader was made to feel stupid or inept.[31]

There are actually a number of forums on the Internet [32] where concerned family members are venting about their loved ones exhibiting bizarre behavior since getting so wrapped up in Access; they fear it is not only a scam but a cult as well.

Alkaline and Ionized Water

Excuse me, exactly *how* does that work? Actually, there are a lot more bogus claims concerning water than just the alkaline/ionized craze, but that seems to be a popular one. One of my own staff members was caught up in it a couple of years ago, and kept bringing me gallons of the stuff to drink. About a year after he was recruited into the company and had spent a small fortune attending sales meetings all over the country, he said "I realize that the fact that it's alkaline doesn't have anything to do with why I'm feeling better. It's just because I'm drinking more water, period."

---

[31] http://dontgotothedarkside.wordpress.com/2011/08/18/hello-world/
Accessed 07/07/2014.

[32] http://www.forum.exscn.net/showthread.php?31933-Help-and-advice-regarding-family-member-joining-Access-Consciousness
Accessed 07/07/2014.

One popular brand of the water filters (and yes, it is an MLM company) sells for about $4000. My husband, who is pretty handy with tools, looked one over and said he could build one with parts from the hardware store for about $45. Why is alkaline water supposedly good for you? The claims are that it will neutralize the effects of acidic foods, and that it's an anti-oxidant. In reality, pure water is neither acidic nor alkaline, nor can it be transformed into either state by electrolysis.

At any rate, the instant you swallow it and it hits the gastric acid in your digestive system, it ceases to be alkaline. There is no scientific evidence that drinking alkaline water has any effect whatsoever on the body.[33]

There is much more water-related pseudoscience and quackery listed **on this website**, which is authored by a retired chemistry professor.[34]

BioMat

I conducted one of my scientific FB polls yesterday; there are several thousand massage therapists on my page, and I asked for people to share their personal opinion about what they thought are the biggest scams and/or weirdest things being sold to massage therapists. The BioMat was the winner, hands-down.

---

[33] **http://www.chem1.com/CQ/ionbunk.html** Accessed 07/01/2014.

[34] **http://www.chem1.com/CQ/index.html** Accessed 07/01/2014.

The BioMat is an item that cashes in on using the term "far-infrared." Far-infrared, for the uninformed, is heat that is emitted by all bodies that have a temperature above absolute zero. At a retail price of $1450 for a massage-table sized mat, that's one expensive heating pad. According to the company's marketing hype, the BioMat emits far-infrared rays, "life-giving" negative ions, and heals you with the amethyst that is embedded in the mat.

I took the time to lie down on one at a convention and I was not impressed. When I asked the woman in the booth to explain to me how it works, she mentioned the far-infrared and the negative ions—but could not tell me what either one of those terms mean! She just knew them as buzzwords to sell the product, and had no actual clue of the definition.

I'm so clever that sometimes I don't understand a single word of what I'm saying.

~ Oscar Wilde

The BioMat website states: *Amethyst healing is an art and practice, done on a metaphysical level that has been re-discovered because of the power of the earth's energies that have been absorbed by these sacred objects. In turn, they inherit vital healing powers for many types of ailments. Amethyst has come to be known as a power crystal with prolific healing powers that can be characterized as purifying, pacifying and transitional. Amethyst has the ability to transform lower energies into higher and acts as a healer at all levels of mind, body, and spirit.*

It further goes on to say *(It will) increase blood circulation, promote perspiration, relieve neuralgia, backaches, and arthritis, and eliminate toxins. The far Infrared rays are good for relaxation, perform an anti-bacterial function and purify the air.*

Exactly *how* does that work? Well, for one thing, if you lay on any heating pad for long enough, you'll probably perspire. I'm afraid that's about it for the good news. The firm that manufactures the BioMat has been called on the carpet by the FDA for their misleading advertising.[35]

There is no scientific evidence that shows any health benefits to be derived from negative ions, and even in the event that there were, they cannot be emitted into the body from an outside source. As for amethysts, they're very pretty, and not very expensive as gemstones go. I own a few impressive specimens myself, bought at rock and mineral shows for as little as $5-10. There is also no evidence of any kind that amethyst can do anything at all to promote health and/or healing of any condition.

Bottom line: you'll get the same exact benefits from a heating pad purchased at Wally World for $25, but hey, it's *your* money. Unless, of course, you're sucking clients into paying to lay on it by promising them health benefits—other than said

[35] **http://www.fda.gov/ICECI/EnforcementActions/WarningLetters/ucm 335214.m** Accessed 07/01/2014.

perspiration. Professional ethics are just plain pesky, aren't they?

Crystal Healing

I love rocks. They're beautiful. They're natural minerals produced by good old Mother Nature (and of course, synthesized fake ones grown in labs are available, too.) I have a rather impressive collection myself. Before the Reformation, I would have slapped a few on your chakras to bring you into balance, or used a nice point to exorcise that negative energy from you, via psychic surgery. Heck, if I had known they existed back then, I might have even bought a BioMat.

No need to throw out your crystal pendant, but don't depend on it to keep you healthy or happy. Feel free to decorate your home or office with your specimens, but don't depend on them to keep your home safe from all harm.

According to the hype on the website of one "crystal healer,"[36] amethyst will cure stomach and liver problems. Emeralds should be used for major illnesses...so if you have cancer, better run out and buy a few carats. Citrine will align your spine. Green fluorite will balance your hormones if you have PMS or you're going through menopause. Putting sodalite next to your computer will protect you from that nasty electromagnetic radiation. Really? Exactly *how* does that work? It doesn't.[37]

---

[36] **http://gems4friends.com/therapeutic-gemstone-properties.html** Accessed 07/01/2014.

There is no evidence anywhere to support any of these claims. They are just made up by people who apparently have a lot of time on their hands. Many books and numerous websites are devoted to the subject. The theory is that crystals have all have their own level of vibration, and that by applying a higher vibration to your diseased body or an object, you can raise that vibration and it will cure what ails you. The website author claimed that carnelian stopped her husband's allergies within 30 seconds. She also claims to have had "profound results," although she doesn't say what kind, with diamond therapy. Poor Elizabeth Taylor. Dripping in diamonds, unarguably the most expensive rock specimens in existence, and she still died from congestive heart failure. I guess that didn't work for her.

It also didn't work in a study conducted by Dr. Christopher French, at Goldsmith's College in London. In a study of 80 people, half received an actual crystal specimen and the other half received cheap fakes. Both groups were given instructions on meditating with the crystal and a booklet containing an explanation of all the sensations they might expect to have while holding the crystal. Only 6 people failed to experience at least one of the sensations. Dr. French's conclusion was that the power of suggestion was responsible and that believers in the paranormal are more susceptible to believing in the power of crystals. [38]

---

[37] **http://www.skepdic.com/crystals.html** Accessed 07/01/2014.

[38] **http://www.telegraph.co.uk/news/uknews/1328277/New-Age-crystal-power-is-all-in-the-mind.html** Accessed 07/07/2014.

Detoxification Cleanses

Real detoxification in our bodies takes place in the liver. The chemical structure of the substances we ingest are modified so they can be filtered by the kidneys, from the blood into the urine, where it is expelled from the body. Metabolic wastes leave our bodies when we urinate, defecate, and perspire. If we accidentally swallow a real toxin, we may get our stomach pumped or have vomiting induced to get rid of it. To hear some people tell it, we're all just one big walking blob of toxins, and we'd best clean that out by doing some type of cleanse. Excuse me, exactly *how* does that work?

"Detox" is a prime example of medical terminology that has been turned into marketing hype, in an attempt to convince consumers that it's a legitimate, science-based product or treatment. On nearly all packaging for "detoxification" cleanses, there is usually no mention of exactly what toxins are supposed to be removed from the body by using the product. It's just a buzzword.

Detox advocates usually focus on the colon. [39] They maintain that some sort of toxic sludge (sometimes called a mucoid plaque) is accumulating in the colon, making it a breeding ground for parasites, *Candida* (yeast) and other nastiness. Fortunately, science tells us otherwise: mucoid plaques and toxic sludge are just a made-up idea to sell detox treatments. Ask any gastroenterologist (who looks inside colons for a living) if they've ever seen one. There isn't a single case that's been documented in the medical literature. Not one.

---

[39] **http://www.sciencebasedmedicine.org/the-detox-scam-how-to-spot-it-and-how-to-avoid-it/** Accessed 07/04/2014.

Detox cleanses range from the simple things you have at home (olive oil and orange juice for a gall bladder cleanse, coffee enemas to clean out the colon) to expensive packaged (and often MLM) products.

On the whole, people aren't stupid, but they're looking for an easy way out, and depending on something that lasts a few days to get rid of a lifetime of abuse or neglect of their bodies. The best way to stay healthy is to follow a good diet, use more calories than you take in by getting plenty of exercise, get plenty of sleep, avoid smoking, avoid abuse of any substances, and in general, take good care of yourself.

If you give up fast food for a week or a month (the average recommended time for a lot of cleanses), give up sugar and/or salt and alcohol, drink more water, exercise more, and generally try to live a more healthy life, you're almost certain to see results in losing weight, feeling better, and looking better, but depending on some kind of cleanse to "detox" you is an exercise in futility.

Detox Foot Pads

Gee whiz, folks, were you paying attention in anatomy class? Exactly *how* does that work?

As I stated above, real detoxification in our bodies takes place in the liver, which modifies the chemical structure of substances so they can be excreted by the kidneys, which act as a filter, from the blood into the urine. Sweat glands in the feet can excrete water and some dissolved substances. However, its minor role in ridding the body of unwanted substances is not changed by applying foot pads. [40]

In April 2008, ABC's "20/20" investigated Kinoki and Avon pads and reported:

- When used overnight, the pads darkened, but dropping distilled water on the pads produced the same dark color.
- Laboratory analysis of pads used by eight volunteers showed no significant evidence of heavy metals or commonly used solvents.
- When asked for tests that would show that their products really work the companies offered no valid scientific studies.

The last bullet is at the real core of the problem with everything mentioned in this book: 1) People are selling something (goods or services). 2) The potential buyer asks how it works—or doesn't even bother to question the authority figure making the claims. 3) The seller cannot produce any

---

[40] **http://www.devicewatch.org/reports/kinoki.shtml** Accessed 07/02/2014.

(truthful) explanation, because there *is* no explanation, other than an unfounded, fantasy-based explanation.

Ear Candling

Some practitioners refer to this as "Hopi Ear Candling." The Biosun company appears to be responsible for that rumor, but according to Vanessa Charles, the public relations officer for the Hopi Cultural Preservation Office, there is absolutely nothing in their history of using ear candling, and it is not a Hopi practice. The Hopi nation would like to have all references to them removed from this procedure.[41]

Proponents of ear candling claim that it creates a low-level vacuum in the ear that will remove ear wax and "debris" from the ear. Gùilty as charged. Ear candling was taught in the massage school I attended—presented, strangely enough, with the class on lymphatic drainage. I did it for years, and I also had it on my menu of services in my business. I removed it as part of the Reformation.

Scientific studies have been conducted that demonstrate that there is no negative pressure created by the burning candles inserted into the ear.

In clinical trials, the results have shown that no wax was removed from the recipient's ear, while wax from the candle was actually deposited in the recipient's ear, in some cases causing damage to the eardrum.

[41] **http://freespace.virgin.net/ahcare.qua/index5.html** Accessed 07/02/2014.

The result of this analysis of clinical trials was that the claimed mechanism by which is works is not verified, and there is no evidence that it is an effective treatment for any condition. [42] Canada actually has legislation prohibiting the importation of ear candles.

Anytime a company makes health-related claims about a product, they are obligated to have that product reviewed by the Food and Drug Administration. 15 candle-makers in the US have been warned by the FDA about making such claims, but they continue to do so, and people continue to use them.

Energy Work

I've discussed that at length at the beginning of this book, but I feel compelled to say more.

I honestly feel it is a losing battle to get anyone who practices energy work to admit that it is synonymous with faith healing. Since my own Reformation, as far as I know, I have never influenced another person's view on the matter. I have witnessed FB groups, where scientists tried to explain some concrete facts to people about energy or other things, and they were attacked and subjected to name-calling, had their credentials questioned, and have been accused of spewing hatred when that is not the case at all. I've dropped out of most of them on account of that. Trying to inspire people to make use of critical thinking is a like trying to herd cats.

---

[42] http://www.ncbi.nlm.nih.gov/pmc/articles/PMC2231549/
Accessed 07/02/2014.

Reiki, Therapeutic Touch®, Healing Touch™ and other practices along that same vein are available in over 800 hospitals in the US. Of course, these same hospitals have religious pastors and chaplains coming in every day, as well, so there's that aspect of it.

Recently, a study was conducted on cultural competency, autonomy, and spiritual conflicts related to reiki/CAM patients in hospitals, focusing on the question, "should patients be informed?"[43] The article abstract points out that many hospitals are offering reiki, but that Catholic hospitals have banned the practice of reiki in their facilities because it conflicts with their religious doctrine. One of the main points of the paper is that in many hospitals, there is no disclosure on the part of the hospital that it is a spiritual practice, and the author examines the ethical concerns and legal implications of such actions. He also offers a proposal of specific information that all practitioners of reiki should disclose to their clients. I'm glad to see I'm not the only one who thinks it's truly unethical not to disclose it.

Energy work can be tested, and has been tested, but it's problematic. When the control group consisted of people receiving no treatment at all, and the reiki group claimed enhanced well-being, it still proved nothing as far as validating reiki, because again, people were having a social visit with a compassionate person who is offering them caring touch. That's been demonstrated time and again. In one experiment where participants who were receiving chemotherapy were randomized to reiki, sham reiki, and standard care, the reiki and the sham reiki group both had better results than the

[43] **http://www.ncbi.nlm.nih.gov/pubmed/24899738** Accessed 07/04/2014.

standard care group, leading to the conclusion that the presence of the nurse offering one-on-one care made a significant difference in how patients felt. [44]

One study was a replication of a study done two decades before in 2003, which had shown that high electromagnetic fields (100nT) emanated from the hands and the hearts of reiki practitioners. [45] The replicated study, performed in 2013 with the much more sophisticated measuring equipment that is available today, showed no electromagnetic measurements above 3nT, clearly demonstrating that the practice of reiki does not appear to produce any routine electromagnetic activity.

A 2008 systematic scientific review of randomized clinical trials of reiki concluded that

...the evidence is insufficient to suggest that reiki is an effective treatment for any condition. The *concept* of ki underlying Reiki is speculative and there is no scientific evidence that it exists.[46]

Both the American Cancer Society and the National Center for Complementary and Alternative medicine have also investigated this notion, and found that there is no clinical or scientific evidence in existence that will support claims that reiki is effective in the treatment of any illness, beyond the placebo effect.

---

[44] http://www.ncbi.nlm.nih.gov/pubmed/21531671 Accessed 07/06/2014.

[45] http://www.ncbi.nlm.nih.gov/pubmed/23210468 Accessed 07/06/2014.

[46] http://www.ncbi.nlm.nih.gov/pubmed/18410352 Accessed 07/06/2014.

Though proper placebo trials of reiki are complicated by design difficulties due to "blinding" requirements, trials conducted with adequate placebo or sham controls have shown no difference between the procedure-treated and the control groups. Even a 2009 review in *The Journal of Alternative and Complementary Medicine* found that

...the serious methodological and reporting limitations of limited existing reiki studies preclude a definitive conclusion on its effectiveness.

Again, the mere presence of a caring person in attendance on someone who is not well, whether they are performing any reiki or not, is enough to produce the same effect of enhanced wellbeing.

The National Certification Board for Therapeutic Massage & Bodywork has page after page of CE classes in energy work listed. Months ago, several other people and I called them out for approving ridiculous classes. When I sent in my list of complaints, I did not even pick on any of the Eastern energy work classes, because their bylaws allow for it. I had a long list of classes that were in actual violation of their own rules, which state that classes on spirituality and religion are not suitable for CE, nor are classes that are based on a product you are selling that a student is obligated to buy in order to participate in the class.

I'd like to state for the record that anyone should feel free to spend their time and money taking any class they choose, even if that's Healing with Leprechauns (I actually did report one called "Healing with the Flower Devas". In case you don't know, deva means "fairy.") That does not, however, mean that our National Certification Board should be giving you credit for taking it. Another class I reported was called "Biblical Anatomy." I haven't attended that one, so I was wondering if it was going to include the particulars of God making woman out of Adam's rib.

Reiki, chakra, and polarity classes abound on the approved CE list. So do classes that are just called "Energy Work/Medicine/Healing," and "Esoteric Healing." I'm looking through their pages right now, and see that "Introduction to a Healing Ministry" has been archived, as has "Reiki with the Angels". Those should have never passed muster to begin with. Neither should "Divine Healer Training," but it's still there. Access Bars® is, too. Numerous crystal healing classes are still allowed, as is "Spiritual Healing Massage". There are also a lot of classes in light therapy, color therapy, and sound therapy. Energy Healing for Bones...excuse me, exactly *how* does that work? If it did work, couldn't we just do away with orthopedic surgeons? I could go on, but that's enough. It's making me ill just to read it.

It's alarming to me that a certification board that should be a hallmark of excellence had allowed things to deteriorate to this level. According to their current president, Dr. Leena Guptha, they have appointed a task force to clean this mess up. When I recently spoke to her about it, she made the comment that "we have a lot of disagreement among the experts on the panel." I'm sure they do. It didn't get in this condition overnight and won't be fixed overnight. Past and current officers of the American Massage Therapy Association practice and teach some of these classes that I'm complaining about. There is support for them at the top of the profession. In reality, there's also a big demand for it, or there wouldn't be so many people teaching it and lining up to take the classes.

The certification boards of the other health care professions do not allow credit for classes in pseudoscience. It does not speak well of massage therapy as a profession that we do.

Personally, I'd like to see some sort of separate credential offered for people who have vowed to uphold an evidence-based practice. I'd like for the medical community to know that not every massage therapist out there is healing with the fairies and claiming to manipulate people's energy with a crystal wand. If medical doctors saw even a tenth of the discussions on some of the FB massage groups, they would never take us seriously enough to refer a patient to any of us.

Flower Essences

Flower essences, the most well-known of which are the Bach flower remedies, are extreme dilutions of flower materials. Edward Bach, the founder, believed that the dew found on flower petals retained the healing properties of the plants. Excuse me, exactly *how* does that work?

There is no doubt that many plants do contain healing properties. Many medicines are in fact derived from plants, including good old aspirin, heart drugs, even cancer-fighting drugs,[47] but the dilution of flower essences is so small that it's doubtful that even one molecule of the plant properties are present in the dilution, which is in a 50:50 solution of brandy and water. The claim is that they are primarily used to treat

---

[47] **http://www.rain-tree.com/plantdrugs.htm#.U7R8qrHeRcg**
Accessed 07/02/2014.

emotional and spiritual maladies, through the "vibrational signature" of the plant.[48]

I suggest you'd probably feel better (and spend less money) if you just have a big snifter of brandy and take time to stop and smell the flowers. Systematic reviews of clinical trials have shown that there is no merit to this therapy other than the placebo effect.

Homeopathy

From Wikipedia:

Homeopathy works by stimulating the body's OWN healing mechanisms, through like for like. A substance that would cause symptoms in a healthy person can be used to cure the same symptoms in a sick person by giving a minute, highly potentised dose of that substance acting as a catalyst to jump start their own healing mechanisms. Every one of us has our own natural innate healing powers. All that is needed is the correct stimulus to kick start it. In healthy people this may just be rest and good food but many people become 'stuck' in their physical, emotional or mental illness and cannot recover. Of course there are different levels of health and the choice of potency given should reflect that. Low potencies are given for very physically ill people and higher for those whose problems are emotional or of the mind. Homeopathy is very successful in treating emotional problems such as stress, anxiety and fears.[49]

---

[48] **http://en.wikipedia.org/wiki/Flower_essence_therapy** Accessed 07/01/2014.

Actually, the laws of chemistry state that there is a limit to the dilution that can be made without losing the original substance altogether. The founder of homeopathy, Samuel Hahnemann, who started formulating his theories in the late 1700s, himself realized that there is virtually no chance that even one molecule of original substance would remain after extreme dilutions. But he believed that the vigorous shaking or pulverizing with each step of dilution leaves behind a "spirit-like" essence—"no longer perceptible to the senses"—which cures by reviving the body's "vital force." Modern proponents assert that even when the last molecule is gone, a "memory" of the substance is retained. This notion is unsubstantiated. Moreover, if it were true, every substance encountered by a molecule of water might imprint an "essence" that could exert powerful (and unpredictable) medicinal effects when ingested by a person.[50]

The evidence does not support that homeopathy is effective for anything, and there has actually been a lot of research conducted on it. Prince Charles (celebrity endorsement of the highest order) has been an advocate of homeopathy, and the NHS in Great Britain has actually covered homeopathy under insurance for years. In 2010, the House of Commons Science and Technology Committee released a 275-page report which reviewed the evidence for homeopathy, and the conclusion was for the NHS to stop funding for it, stating that it doesn't work; it can't work, and amounts to little more than witchcraft. This spurred some of the biggest homeopathy companies to re-

---

[49] http://rationalwiki.org/wiki/Wiki4CAM:_Myths_about_homeopathy
Accessed 07/04/2014.

[50] http://www.quackwatch.com/01QuackeryRelatedTopics/homeo.html
Accessed 07/04/2014.

label their products as "confectionary." Nice word for a sugar-pill placebo.

Homeopathic remedies have also been investigated by the FDA in the US. During one investigation, *"the investigator also observed for Batch #36659 that one out of every six bottles did not receive the dose of active homeopathic drug solution due to the wobbling and vibration of the bottle assembly during filling of the active ingredient. The active ingredient was instead seen dripping down the outside of the vial assembly. Your firm lacked controls to ensure that the active ingredient is delivered to every bottle."*

One in six bottles didn't get their dose of nothing, I mean "active ingredient." Homeopaths did not seem to notice this manufacturing defect.[51]

---

[51] **http://www.sciencebasedmedicine.org/homeopathys-recent-woes/** Accessed 07/04/2014.

Ionic Foot Baths

This was the second most popular answer on my FB poll about scams.

Take a tub of water, add two low-current electrodes and some salt to enhance conductivity, place your feet in them for a few minutes (you may want to muscle-test to find out exactly how long you should perform this ritual), and presto! All those nasty toxins will leave your body. The proof is in the discolored water, right?

Wrong.

The only thing the discolored water proves is that iron is corroding off of the electrodes during the process of electrolysis. The water will turn brown whether your feet, a zucchini, or absolutely nothing for that matter, is put in the water.[52]

Many massage therapists, chiropractors, and other practitioners have added this to their menu of services. When these machines first came on the market, they were selling for over $1000. You can now purchase one as cheaply as $100 on e-bay, and people commonly charge from $40 up for having their client sit there soaking their feet while they go on about other business, so it's a definite money-maker...if you want to make your money in an unscrupulous fashion.

---

[52] **http://syndicatednews.net/detox-foot-spa-bath-is-a-scam-and-hoax-heres-why/** Accessed 07/01/2014.

Juice

That's a really generic term, on purpose. There are too many name-brands out there to list them, but some of the more popular are Noni Juice, MonaVie, Xango Juice, Gogi Berry Juice, Acai Berry Juice, and Aloe Vera Juice. These various companies claim that their products are effective treatments for arthritis, slowing down the aging process, curing diabetes, helping vision problems, getting rid of cancer, AIDS, and heart disease, among other things. Excuse me, exactly *how* does that work?

I am not saying that juice is a bad thing. I am saying that if I'm going to pay $25 or more for a bottle of juice, it better come with a cork and a nice vintage.

The buzzword surrounding all these juices is "anti-oxidants." Several of these companies also use the buzzword "ORAC" (Oxygen Radical Absorbance Capacity), which is a scientific test meant to measure anti-oxidant capacities of foods, and is also frequently used with essential oils. According to MonaVie's ORAC score, you'd have to drink 9 ounces of their juice to get the same ORAC found in one apple—and 9 ounces of their juice comes at a cost of over $16. [53]

Berries are in fact full of anti-oxidants; so are pomegranates, mangosteens, leafy green vegetables, and prunes, among other foods. What makes a bottle of one of these high-priced labels any more valuable than the blueberry juice that you can buy in the grocery store for less than $5, or better yet, buy the blueberries and juice your own? Absolutely nothing.

---

[53] **http://www.juicescam.com/** Accessed 07/06/2014.

Most of these juices are sold through multi-level-marketing companies. Some of them come in fancy wine bottles with snazzy-looking labels, and the health claims they make are ridiculous and even dangerous...I've heard horror stories from people that even their family doctor was selling MLM juice and claiming it would help their cancer.

In looking through some of the forums on the Internet about juices, one woman who sells a popular MLM juice added insult to injury when she said "I don't sell it to everyone. I muscle test them first to see if their body really needs it." I'm so glad to hear it. Not!

Many of these expensive juices are full of nothing more than a small amount of whatever miracle ingredient they're touting, with a bigger amount of apple or grape juice for fillers. Labels list ingredients with the highest amount of ingredients listed first. Check out that expensive bottle of acai berry or pomegranate juice and see how far down on the label the pomegranate actually appears, and you probably won't buy any more of it. In the case of MonaVie, which claims to be made from acai berries as their big selling point, acai berries actually only account for 2% of the juice.

Juicing is a different thing altogether, and I am certainly not averse to people juicing their own fruits and vegetables, which many people don't get enough of in their diets. It will be much cheaper for you to juice your own than it will be for you to pay a ridiculous amount of money for what amounts to a bottle of over-priced snake oil. Or snake *juice*.

Oil Pulling

Oil pulling is an Ayurvedic practice that involves putting sesame oil or another oil into your mouth and swishing it around for 10-20 minutes. Proponents claim that it can reduce cavities, cure or prevent gum disease, reduce bacteria in the mouth, and that all-important phrase—detoxify your body.

Swishing any substance around in your mouth—like plain old water—will have some effect of dislodging food particles from the mouth, so it's beneficial in that respect. As far as removing toxins from your body, excuse me, exactly *how* does that work?

Swishing sesame oil around in the mouth for that long causes it to emulsify and turn into a soap-like substance—think scrubbing bubbles. But it's *oil*. It's coating your mouth and your teeth with *oil*.

One abstract on PubMed attributes recurrent lipoid pneumonia to oil pulling. Lipoid pneumonia is a chemical lung disease caused by aspirating (breathing in) small amounts of oil. The long duration of mouth swishing with oil recommended by oil pulling advocates may increase the risk of lipoid pneumonia as a complication. This is a good reminder that no matter how "natural" and "ancient" a treatment is, we should not assume it is entirely without risk.[54]

---

[54] http://www.ncbi.nlm.nih.gov/pubmed/24429325 Accessed 07/04/2014.

Tuning Forks

As a musician, I'm quite familiar with tuning forks. I also availed myself with a session of tuning fork "healing" about ten years ago, to see what all the fuss was about.

The premise behind it is this: *Like adjusting a piano, your body can be tuned to achieve optimal physical balance. Tapping two BioSonic tuning forks will instantaneously alter your body's biochemistry and bring your nervous system, muscle tone and organs into harmonic balance.[55]*

Excuse me, exactly *how* does that work? I can use a tuning fork to *tell me* that my instrument is out of tune, but I must still make the adjustments to the strings manually in order to bring it back into tune. The tuning fork is not going to magically perform that process for me. It would be nice and time-saving if it did.

From the BioSonic website, a description of one set of forks: BioSonics Asteroid Tuning Fork Set, which sells for $87.98.

Asteroids are like muses that come into our lives. Asteroid tuning forks are playful and designed to create a sonic space that wakes us up and motivates our creativity and sense of adventure. If you are excited about something and waiting for a muse to visit then BioSonic asteroid tuning forks will attract your muse.

If I need my muse, I'll call and ask him to come over.

---

[55] **http://www.skepdic.com/vibrationalmedicine.html** Accessed 07/02/2014.

If you'll lay out $299.00, you can get the Planetary Set, which brings new dimensions to your Astrology readings, enhance bodywork and acupuncture sessions, or use for personal meditation and growth.

Yes, music is soothing. It may have a calming effect on you to hear a pleasant note, but it is not going to suddenly bring your body into balance. There is no scientific evidence to support that the body or anything in it, including your cells and your organs, has a certain vibration, or that said vibration can be changed by the application of tuning forks.

Tuning forks do have medical and scientific applications. Quartz tuning forks are commonly used in the branch of science known as microscopy, as a physical probe to help create images of a surface.[56] The intent is not to effect any change on the surface, but merely to obtain an image of the surface. If the tuning fork was creating any kind of change, it would not be useful for that purpose. Tuning forks are also used to assess hearing. Notice I said *assess*, not cure. If tuning forks could actually restore hearing to a deaf person, they'd be used for that purpose. In fact, of the 85 studies indexed on PubMed that refer to tuning forks, all are in the context of their use in scientific imaging and measurement, not in any use for healing anything.

Tuning forks *are* useful, for the purposes they are intended for. Changing the vibration of human tissue is not one of them.

---

[56] **http://en.wikipedia.org/wiki/Scanning_probe_microscopy**
Accessed 07/04/2014.

Vibrational Medicine

That's rather a catch-all term that can encompass energy work, or anything in which the "healer" is claiming to detect, or change, the "vibration" of the human body in order to facilitate healing. That would include the tuning forks mentioned above, and the crystal healing, among other things.

Dr. Albert Abrams (1863-1924), the "dean of twentieth century charlatans." [57] Abrams claimed that he was able to detect distinct energies or vibrations_(radiation) being emitted from healthy and diseased tissue in all living things. He invented devices that allegedly could measure this energy (vibration, radiation) and he created a system for evaluating vibrations as signs of health or disease. As I stated in the previous section on tuning forks, there is no scientific evidence to support that the body or anything in it, including your cells and your organs, has a certain vibration, or that said vibration can be changed by the application of some sort of device.

While all modern tests have shown that Abrams' devices, and similar inventions by those who have come after him, fail to do what they say they are going to do, proponents claim that the healer must have paranormal powers in order to pick up the measurements. I guess that means you'll have to run out and find a psychic or medium if you want an accurate test.

Quackery involving all kinds of machinery and "biofeedback" software that claims to detect and cure all kinds of illnesses, from allergies to cancer, by vibration or frequencies is running rampant. Supporters argue that medical science just hasn't

---

[57] **http://www.skepdic.com/radionics.html** Accessed 07/05/2014.

caught up yet. I say that medical science would be the first to use it, if it actually worked. That's why we have x-rays, CAT scans, MRIs, EEGs, microscopy, and the like. Those proved to be capable of detecting and/or measuring something and were put into use. If this actually worked at measuring anything, it would be put into use, as well.

There could be a cool million dollars at stake here! James Randi, known around the world as a magician and escape artist, has for years offered a cash prize to anyone who could offer proof of the paranormal. Back in 1964, when he first made the offer, it was $1000, but he is now offering $1 million. In addition, there are skeptic societies all over the Internet that offer monetary prizes of varying sizes to anyone who can back up their claims under controlled conditions. *Scientific American* magazine has offered a cash prize to anyone who could produce an authentic spirit photograph since 1922. So far, no winners.

Randi's website is a hoot...page after page of some of the things people have tried to prove in order to win the $1 million and failed, or who withdrew their application altogether when they saw that anything they propose must be done under controlled conditions so fakery and bias can't enter into it. One tuning fork healer withdrew her application.

One homeopath withdrew his application to prove he could cure sick people with homeopathy, when the Randi Foundation informed him that they would not approve of a test protocol where people were prohibited from getting regular healthcare if they wanted it. They asked him to instead identify a bottle as containing either plain water or a homeopathic remedy, and he withdrew his application. For crying out loud, he had a 50/50 chance of getting it right. Various "healers", psychics, people who claim they can diagnose someone just by looking at their photograph, dowsers, animal communicators, telepaths and many others have tried. Randi still has his million dollars.

Again, if people ask "What's the harm?" the harm is in people believing in a cure that doesn't exist.

Consegrity® is a type of faith healing, described as energy medicine, developed by a doctor, Mary Lynch, who died in 2012, and a massage therapist, Debra Harrison, who died in 2005 while she was being treated by Lynch. [58] She died from untreated diabetes. Harrison's mother, who also was a follower of Consegrity®, refused medical care until it was too late, and she died from cancer. Harrison's family was accused of causing her death with their "negative energy" because they had begged her to give up on the faith healing and seek medical care. That's the logic of those who try to rationalize the failure of a magical therapy. The media hype of Consegrity®, which is now out of business said:

Consegrity works with the electromagnetic, vibrational systems of the body by reflecting/mirroring in a way that supports neutralizing the disruption, thereby grounding the overload along fluid dynamics restoring balance at the level of the cause bridging management of healthcare and supporting optimum, viable health.

---

[58] **http://www.skepdic.com/consegrity.html** Accessed 07/07/2012.

Sounds like that statement came directly from the **New Age Bullshit Generator**[59], which I think is one of the most hilarious things on the Internet.

Lynch and Harrison's question to people was "How do you choose to feel?" Apparently, these two "healers" couldn't heal themselves. Maybe they had negative energy.

Weight Loss Scams

I don't think anyone can match Dr. Oz for the sheer number of weight loss scams he has touted on his television show. The Cult of Oz has gone running out and bought them all in their desperation to lose weight. [60]

Sen. Claire McCaskill, chairwoman of the Subcommittee on Consumer Protection, Product Safety and Insurance, led the panel that on Tuesday looked at false advertising for weight loss products. Subcommittee members took issue with assertions that Oz has made on his show about products that don't have a lot of scientific evidence to back them up, such as green coffee beans.

"The scientific community is almost monolithic against you in terms of the efficacy of the three products you called 'miracles,' " said McCaskill, a Missouri Democrat. She said she was discouraged by the "false hope" his rhetoric gives viewers and

---

[59] **http://sebpearce.com/bullshit/** Accessed 07/11/2014.

[60] **http://www.cnn.com/2014/06/17/health/senate-grills-dr-oz/** Accessed 07/05/2014

questioned his role "intentional or not, in perpetuating these scams."

"I don't get why you need to say this stuff when you know it's not true. When you have this amazing megaphone, why would you cheapen your show? ... With power comes a great deal of responsibility."

There are literally thousands of bogus weight loss supplements on the market, and most of them are expensive and useless. There are also all kinds of body wraps, thermal sauna suits, weight loss belts, earrings that supposedly perform auricular acupuncture, not to mention weird exercise contraptions, like standing on a vibrating platform and waiting for your fat to just vibrate right off you.

I've been overweight for a long time. I've tried many of them myself, and literally dozens of weird diets, too. I know in my heart of hearts that the only way to lose those extra pounds is to eat sensibly and exercise. There's no magic pill, and yet, that's what we hear constantly from the companies who are marketing them. I know better, but I've been sucked right in, along with millions of others who need to lose weight. We're bombarded with ads and infomercials and celebrities saying "This is IT! It's miraculous! I lost 30 pounds in one month!"

Dr. Oz touted one supplement, Garcinia cambogia, with a big screen in the background saying "No Diet. No Exercise. No Effort." Excuse me, exactly *how* does that work? It doesn't. Not only is that fudging on the truth, it's just an outright lie.

The Federal Trade Commission has compiled a list of seven statements that experts say simply cannot be true, when it comes to advertising of weight loss products. [61] They're called the "7 Gut Check Claims" and were actually created by the FTC for media outlets to use as a litmus test before running any advertisements for weight loss products. Of course, the mighty dollar wins out consistently over any scruples when it comes to selling advertising.

Here's the Gut Check list:

1. causes weight loss of two pounds or more a week for a month or more without dieting or exercise;
2. causes substantial weight loss no matter what or how much the consumer eats;
3. causes permanent weight loss even after the consumer stops using product;
4. blocks the absorption of fat or calories to enable consumers to lose substantial weight;
5. safely enables consumers to lose more than three pounds per week for more than four weeks;
6. causes substantial weight loss for all users; or
7. causes substantial weight loss by wearing a product on the body or rubbing it into the skin.

Some companies get around the Gut Check list by just making variations on the statements, but the bottom line is always the same...there is nothing out there that will cause you to lose weight, and enable you to sustain that loss, unless you are making the effort. You should run, not walk, from any product that claims you don't have to make any changes in your

---

[61] http://www.business.ftc.gov/documents/0492-gut-check-reference-guide-media-spotting-false-weight-loss-claims Accessed 07/05/2014.

lifestyle, or any product that makes claims of a dramatic weight loss in a short period of time.

There are some products on the market that are legitimate "fat-blockers," that will prevent your body from absorbing fat. These aren't good for several reasons. We all actually need *some* fat in our bodies. In order for a fat-blocker to work, you would still have to be on a reduced-calorie diet. And if you read the labels, you'll see that these products have some lovely side effects, such as causing extreme flatulence and anal leakage...and yet, people line up to take them. Along with the fat-blockers, I've recently seen advertisements for "sugar-blockers," telling you that you can still have your cake and eat it, too, with no worries of gaining weight. That would be nice if it was true, but it isn't.

Weight loss is an internal metabolic process, so weight loss claims for body wraps, lotions, potions, patches, earrings, belts, bracelets, or anything you put on your skin is not going to cause a substantial weight loss.

There are things on the market such as wraps and diuretics that can cause a temporary loss of excess fluids in the body. There are other products, and diets, out there that are intended to send your body into a state of ketosis, which forces the body to burn fats instead of carbohydrates, which are normally the body's fuel.

Weight loss that is supervised by a physician may sometimes include shots or supplements intended to act as an appetite suppressant. In extreme cases, people sometimes opt for bariatric surgery to lose weight. Even having a surgery is no guarantee that the weight you lose will stay off permanently, unless you abide by the required commitment to change your eating and exercise habits.

There's no one diet that will work for everyone. In order to lose weight, an obese child will require a different diet than an obese middle-aged person. A diabetic requires a different diet than someone who isn't diabetic. Pregnant women have different dietary needs than women who aren't pregnant.

There seems to be almost as many people following dietary rules as there obese people: people who are vegan or vegetarian, people who are lactose-intolerant, people who are eating gluten-free, people who avoid certain foods for religious reasons or because they have allergies. Even a vegetarian could be fat or unhealthy. There's just no one-size-fits-all.

Remember the food pyramid that the USDA (United States Department of Agriculture) used to have? That's now been replaced by MyPlate,[62] depicting a plate and a glass that's divided into 5 sections. It's approximately 30% grains, 30%

[62] **http://www.cnpp.usda.gov/MyPlate.htm** Accessed 07/05/2014.

[63] **http://healthyeating.sfgate.com/body-process-fruit-sugars-same-way-refined-sugar-8174.html** Accessed 07/05/2014.

vegetables, 20% fruits and 20% protein. A separate small cup represents dairy, which they recommend consuming as low-fat, 1% milk, and foods like yogurt.

In reality, the sugars found in fruit are the same as those found in refined sugar, and the only real difference is the rate at which they are metabolized. Refined sugar is sucrose[63], which is made up of glucose and fructose, and is metabolized very quickly. Fruit, depending on the type, may be any combination of sucrose, glucose, and fructose, and the fact that it contains fiber is the reason it metabolizes at a slower rate, and doesn't cause the "insulin spike" that people often get from eating candy. If the energy from that chocolate bar isn't used immediately, it turns into fat. Besides fiber, fruit also contains beneficial anti-oxidants, vitamins, minerals, and phytonutrients.

The bottom line is back up from the table and get up and *do something* if you want to lose weight. In spite of Dr. Oz and all those late-night infomercials, and all the companies out there who'd like to take our money for magic weight loss, it just isn't going to happen, no matter how much we'd like to think otherwise.

Those Pesky Ethics

Ethics is knowing the difference in what you have the right to do and what is right to do.

~Potter Stewart

What does the Code of Ethics have to do with any of this? Plenty, that's what. If you are providing services, and/or goods to consumers, then pay attention. Every regulated state has a Code of Ethics, and if you're a licensed practitioner, you have agreed to uphold it. Since those vary somewhat, I'm going to draw on the Code from the National Certification Board of Therapeutic Massage & Bodywork[64], because in spite of any other shortcomings I may perceive them to have, I believe they have the finest Code in the profession. They go way beyond what most other organizations or boards spell out, and I think that's good.

If you're practicing in an unregulated state, you're not legally bound to abide by the Code. However, I hope that from a standpoint of someone who is viewing and holding themselves out to be a professional therapist, you would agree to abide by it anyway. People have different ideas about what's morally right or wrong. One person may think prostitution, or gambling, or abortion is fine, while someone else thinks it's

---

[64] **http://www.ncbtmb.org/code-ethics** Accessed 07/05/2014.

wrong. What's illegal is not necessarily immoral, and vice versa...that's why all licensed professions have a Code of Ethics that licensees agree to abide by.

My thoughts, which are mostly questions to ask of yourself, on follow the statements and are written in italics. My hope is that you will examine your conscience and see if you are making a good-faith effort to abide by the Code. My hope is that instead of blindly following the leader, or blindly accepting whatever you've been taught, that you will question things for yourself, that you'll raise your hand and say "Excuse me, exactly *how* does that work?" My hope is that if someone ever asks you the question, "Excuse me, exactly *how* does that work?" whether it's a client you're providing treatment or selling products to, or a student you are teaching, you will keep this Code foremost in mind when you are giving them an answer.

Code of Ethics

I. Have a sincere commitment to provide the highest quality of care to those who seek their professional services.

Does providing the "highest quality of care" include being truthful with our clients about what we are doing, and how it works? Or does it mean we can just do or sell them anything, regardless of whether there is any sound basis for it working or not? What about when there's direct evidence that it doesn't work beyond placebo effect?

II. Represent their qualifications honestly, including education and professional affiliations, and provide only those services that they are qualified to perform.

This means what it says. Unless you are qualified to act as a physician, psychologist, registered nutritionist or dietician, or have the credentials of any other licensed profession, you should not be providing those services.

III. Accurately inform clients, other health care practitioners, and the public of the scope and limitations of their discipline.

Do you know what your scope of practice is? Many people don't, because they haven't bothered to read the Practice Act in their state. There are limitations on what we're allowed to do, and rightly so. This goes back to the statement above in II, about only providing services you are truly qualified to perform.

IV. Acknowledge the limitations of and contraindications for massage and bodywork and refer clients to appropriate health professionals.

It's careless and dangerous to act as if we know more than the doctor does. Don't allow ego to take over to the detriment of your client's health by thinking you know better.

V. Provide treatment only where there is reasonable expectation that it will be advantageous to the client.

If the natural laws of the universe, anatomy, biology, chemistry, physics, and/or physiology overwhelmingly supports the view that is opposite to yours, are you really abiding by this part of the Code? Well, even the placebo effect has been shown to be beneficial, but where do you draw the line?

VI. Consistently maintain and improve professional knowledge and competence, striving for professional excellence through regular assessment of personal and professional strengths and weaknesses and through continued education training.

If you're one of those people who resent taking continuing education because you know it all, that's a professional weakness of the worst sort. A good mentor can help you recognize your strengths, build on them, and help you overcome weaknesses.

VII. Conduct their business and professional activities with honesty and integrity, and respect the inherent worth of all persons.

The same sermon I've been preaching throughout this book: be honest with people about what you're doing. Be honest about it if you're offering something that must be taken on faith. Integrity means full disclosure to clients.

VIII. Refuse to unjustly discriminate against clients and/or health professionals.

Hopefully, no one is discriminating against clients because of their race, religion, gender, sexual orientation, ethnicity, or other reason. Prejudice is an ugly thing. Bad-mouthing doctors and traditional medicine isn't apt to win you any referrals.

IX. Safeguard the confidentiality of all client information, unless disclosure is requested by the client in writing, is medically necessary, is required by law, or necessary for the protection of the public.

If you believe a client is a danger to themselves or others, that should be reported to the proper authorities. Otherwise, their information is sacred. Sharing the names of your celebrity clients on social media is unacceptable, but I see that happening all the time.

X. Respect the client's right to treatment with informed and voluntary consent. The certified practitioner will obtain and record the informed consent of the client, or client's advocate, before providing treatment. This consent may be written or verbal.

Prime example of why it's unethical to perform energy work on clients who do not believe in it and have not requested it. It may be that they reject it for religious reasons, and if they haven't given informed consent, then you shouldn't do it.

XI. Respect the client's right to refuse, modify or terminate treatment regardless of prior consent given.

If a client becomes uncomfortable at any time with any action that happens in the therapeutic relationship, they have every right to withdraw their consent.

XII. Provide draping and treatment in a way that ensures the safety, comfort and privacy of the client.

We are the only profession, other than doctors and nurses,that put our hands on unclothed people. They need to feel secure and comfortable at all times. Careless draping and too casual of an attitude, even when there was no evil intent, has cost many a therapist their license and their livelihood.

XIII. Exercise the right to refuse to treat any person or part of the body for just and reasonable cause.

That little voice is inside your head for a reason. Listen to it. If you feel hesitant or uncomfortable about providing services to someone, then you shouldn't do it.

XIV. Refrain, under all circumstances, from initiating or engaging in any sexual conduct, sexual activities, or sexualizing behavior involving a client, even if the client attempts to sexualize the relationship unless a pre-existing relationship exists between an applicant or a practitioner and the client prior to the applicant or practitioner applying to be certified by NCBTMB.

There is a power differential in every therapeutic relationship, and it's in favor of the provider. The burden is on us to behave ethically and professionally, and to either turn the tide or terminate the relationship immediately if the client is the one in violation.

XV. Avoid any interest, activity or influence which might be in conflict with the practitioner's obligation to act in the best interests of the client or the profession.

Big example: recruiting clients to buy something we are selling, by telling them that they need it, or getting them into the MLM we're involved in. That immediately places you in a dual relationship, which is not a good thing. Making money off of clients, over and above charging them our normal and customary fee, is unethical.

XVI. Respect the client's boundaries with regard to privacy, disclosure, exposure, emotional expression, beliefs and the client's reasonable expectations of professional behavior. Practitioners will respect the client's autonomy.

The client should always feel safe and secure in the relationship they have with you. If emotional expression takes a turn for the worse and the client experiences emotional release on the table, just be present for them, ask if they want to continue with the session, and avoid the urge to start counseling them.

XVII. Refuse any gifts or benefits that are intended to influence a referral, decision or treatment, or that are purely for personal gain and not for the good of the client.

Some states also have statutes that prohibit any type of reward for referrals, including adding time on to a session or giving a free massage when someone refers x number of people. Hopefully, people are referring to you because they believe you're a great therapist, not because you are offering them a reward to do so.

XVIII. Follow the NCBTMB Standards of Practice, this Code of Ethics, and all policies, procedures, guidelines, regulations, codes, and requirements promulgated by the National Certification Board for Therapeutic Massage & Bodywork. *The Code and the Standards are thorough and professional, and available as a reference for all, certificant or not.*

We're Never Going to Agree

People will generally accept facts as truth only if the facts agree with what they already believe.

~Andy Rooney

While I would be thrilled to know that even one person embraced evidence-based, or evidence-informed, as some people prefer to say, practice on account of what I've written here, I don't expect it to happen. If even one person who is practicing energy work informed the client that it is a faith healing practice, I'd be thrilled, but I'm not sitting around waiting for it to happen.

The FB arguments will still go on (albeit without my participation). Practitioners will still be performing things on people without telling them what it is. They'll still be selling people time on their BioMat or their detox foot bath, without being able to explain to people how it works—because it doesn't work. People will continue to give advice that they aren't qualified to give. Why should I care?

I do care. I would like to see massage therapy accepted as mainstream medical care, available to all, whether they have insurance coverage or not, and see it covered when they do. I would like for physicians to have respect for us, and to view us as a valuable part of the health care team. As long as we're known for embracing pseudoscience, I don't think it will happen.

I've probably made a few more enemies here, but that's okay. I feel better for having explained my position and clearing up some of the misconceptions about what I believe. I don't disown people or unfriend them on my social media sites for disagreeing with me.

I don't think any holistic practitioner sets out on their career thinking "Let me see how much money I can make by offering fake treatments." I think the majority are genuinely caring people who just want to help people. I also believe that many are guilty of the same blind acceptance I was, and that it doesn't even occur to them that they're learning or using something that is based on faith and not fact.

If even one person, when they're about to purchase some gizmo, pay for a faith healing, or they're sitting in a class, raises their hand and says "Excuse me, exactly *how* does that work?" then I've accomplished what I want to do, which is to make people think.

Just like I have friends that don't share my politics, my religion (or lack of it), or other belief systems, I have friends that practice or embrace the things I've talked about in this book. I don't disown them on account of it, and they haven't disowned me, at least my true friends haven't.

Feel free to connect with me on FB, Twitter, LinkedIn, and YouTube. You can email me at **laura@lauraallenmt.com**

If you're going to send me hate mail defending your modality, product or treatment, just be sure that you answer the question, *"Excuse me, exactly how does that work?"*

About the Author

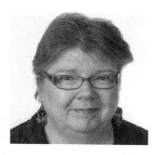

Laura Allen is a massage therapist, clinic owner, educator, author, and blogger. She resides in the mountains of Western North Carolina with her husband Champ, and their two rescued dogs, Queenie and Fido. She is a musician and singer/songwriter and enjoys reading English and Irish literature.

Other Books by Laura Allen:

A Massage Therapist's Guide to Business

Manual for Massage Therapy Educators (*co-authored with Ryan Hoyme*)

One Year to a Successful Massage Therapy Practice

Plain & Simple Guide to Therapeutic Massage & Bodywork Examinations

The Days Still Left

Nothin' Fancy: Good Food and a Few Funny Stories

Made in the USA
Monee, IL
13 February 2022

91232948R00075